Medical Aspects of the Imported Fire Ant

Robert B. Rhoades, M.D.

A University of Florida Book
The University Presses of Florida
Gainesville / 1977

Library of Congress Cataloging in Publication Data

Rhoades, Robert B 1942–
Medical aspects of the imported fire ant.

"A University of Florida book."
1. Fire ants—Venom—Physiological effect.
2. Allergy. 3. Fire ants. I. Title. [DNLM:
1. Ants. QX565 R474m]
RC598.F57R45 615.9'42 77–1736
ISBN 0–8130–0559–0

TYPOGRAPHY BY CANON GRAPHICS, TALLAHASSEE, FLORIDA
PRINTED BY STORTER PRINTING COMPANY, GAINESVILLE, FLORIDA

This book is dedicated to those who influenced my life greatly: my parents; my wife; and my teachers, Drs. Gerold L. Schiebler, Andrew E. Lorincz, and Heinz J. Wittig.

Thanks go to Drs. William Buren and Murray Blum for advice and inspiration and to Darryl Kalof, Gerald Kivett, and Sandra Barnawell for much hard work and technical support.

CONTENTS

1

THE FASCINATING WORLD OF ANTS

The Japanese ideograph for ant is a composite of the characters for "insect . . . unselfishness . . . justice . . . and courtesy" (1).

As one who entered the world of ant-watching through a clinical interest in patients hypersensitive to fire ant stings (2), it has quickly become clear to me how people can spend their lives as ardent and enthusiastic ant-watchers. It is a fascinating and incredible world of "science faction."

Suppose you were to pick up a science fiction book about a Martian creature, an armor-plated monster that would fight on when cut in half, could walk up a 90° grade on a smooth surface while carrying a load several times its own weight, and was capable of smelling a CO_2 or vapor gradient, of seeing in the ultraviolet spectrum, and of "seeing" the plane of polarized light. You might say this is interesting but a bit farfetched. If you were then told that this creature's armor was made of polysaccharide, that it had a brain smaller than the head of a pin yet could do the equivalent of integral calculus, that it could sense and orient in a magnetic field, learn rapidly how to get through a maze, and follow a chemical trail via the directional sensing and integration of chemical gradients present in picamolar amounts, you might well say that this was too improbable a creature to hold your interest. Yet, all of the above facts have been scientifically observed and documented in the ant.

The success of the ant is best expressed in this quotation from Edward Wilson's excellent book *The Insect Societies*:

> On several counts ants can be regarded as the premier social insects. They are the most widely distributed of the major eusocial groups, ranging from the arctic tree line south to

Tierra del Fuego, to the tip of South Africa, and to Tasmania, and occurring on virtually every oceanic island between Iceland and the Aleutians in the north and Tristan da Cunha and Campbell in the south. They are numerically the most abundant of social insects. At any given moment there are at least 10^{15} living ants on the earth, assuming that C. B. Williams (1964) is correct in estimating a total of 10^{18} individual insects—and taking 0.1 percent as a conservative estimate of the proportion made up of ants. The ants contain a greater number of known genera and species than all other eusocial groups combined (3).

The adaptability and specialization of the ant is extreme—some are primarily seed storers (harvester ants), and some rely entirely on "honeydew" (the ants' "national" dish, so to speak), the sugar-containing secretions of homopterous insects such as aphids. The degree of specialization is such that the ants actually "corral" these "cows" (aphids) in or near the nest area, raise and protect them, "put them out to pasture" onto plants, and then collect the honeydew.[1] Farming has been refined in a totally different direction by several *Atta* species who, rather than collect seeds or keep "cows," have become fungus farmers, carefully preparing an appropriate medium for the mold-like fungus, maintaining a pure culture of this mold, and eating only tiny swellings on the hyphae, in a truly symbiotic relationship. There are even species that specialize in making war and taking slaves (i.e., the Amazon ants, *Polyergus* spp.) (7). They have sickle-shaped mandibles and are incapable of excavating their own nests or gathering food. Therefore, they subsist by raiding other ant colonies and capturing brood from them. They are totally dependent for minute-to-minute care on the slave workers they rear from this brood. In *Teleutomyrmex schneideri* the queen has become a totally dependent louse-like parasite, her body modified for riding on the back of her host queen (3). There are many other instances of mutualism or symbiosis, such as the relationships between the fungus-growing ants and their fungus or among certain tropical parabiotic species—pairs of distantly related species which, nevertheless, nest together and trail together. Others include cer-

1. Gall insect-keeping by *Solenopsis* species has been described by Wilson (5) and Whitcomb (6).

tain tropical ants and specific plants which depend entirely on the ants for pollination and in return supply nectar. There is the fascinating relationship between a group of plants known as myrmecophytes and their resident ants; the plant accommodates the ants by providing special lodging and special food, while the ants protect the plant from predators and competitors, including other plants. Ants are found from the treetops (certain arboreal species) to underground (certain subterranean species) (3, 4). Their vision ranges from that of the larged-eyed fire ant, or the tree dweller (ex. *Pseudomyrmex* spp.), to the totally blind army ant.

The history of the ants is an ancient one. They are presumed to have arisen from the nonsocial Tiphiid wasps over 100 million years ago. As they evolved from this primitive nonsocial ancestor, their socialization became more efficient, and they became progressively more successful.

From the standpoint of hypersensitivity reactions to ants in the United States, the discussion quickly focuses on one group of ants, the genus *Solenopsis*, or fire ants. Within this genus, the species of clinical significance is *S. invicta*, which is the major representative of the so-called imported fire ant (3). This species is responsible for more than 95 percent of the clinical problems. Therefore we will use the fire ant as our prototype and then discuss variations from this model. Allergic reactions can be caused by other ant species (8–10), but such reactions are rare.

The Fire Ant Group

Solenopsis richteri Forel.—This is the black imported fire ant whose homeland is Uruguay and eastern Argentina. It was imported to the Mobile, Alabama, area about 1918 or perhaps earlier, and still exists in the United States in only one region, an elongated area from Pontatuck to Meridian in Mississippi, with extensions into northwestern Alabama (Fig. 1). It is usually distinguishable to the naked eye by its black or brownish-black color and the large yellow spot on the gaster (abdomen) of larger workers. It constructs large, often conical, mounds.

Solenopsis invicta Buren.—The red imported fire ant's home is the State of Mato Grosso, Brazil, but its range extends along the Guaporé River to the north, and south along the Paraguay River to northern Argentina (Fig. 2). It was imported to the Mobile,

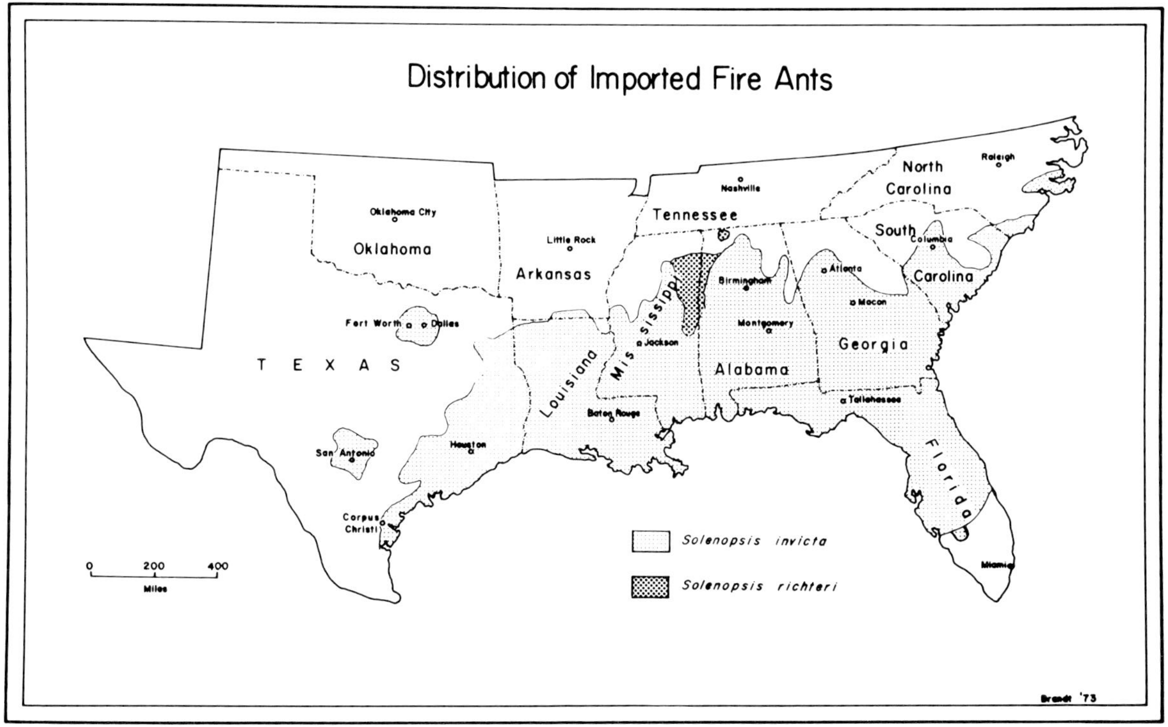

Figure 1. Distribution of the imported fire ant in the United States.

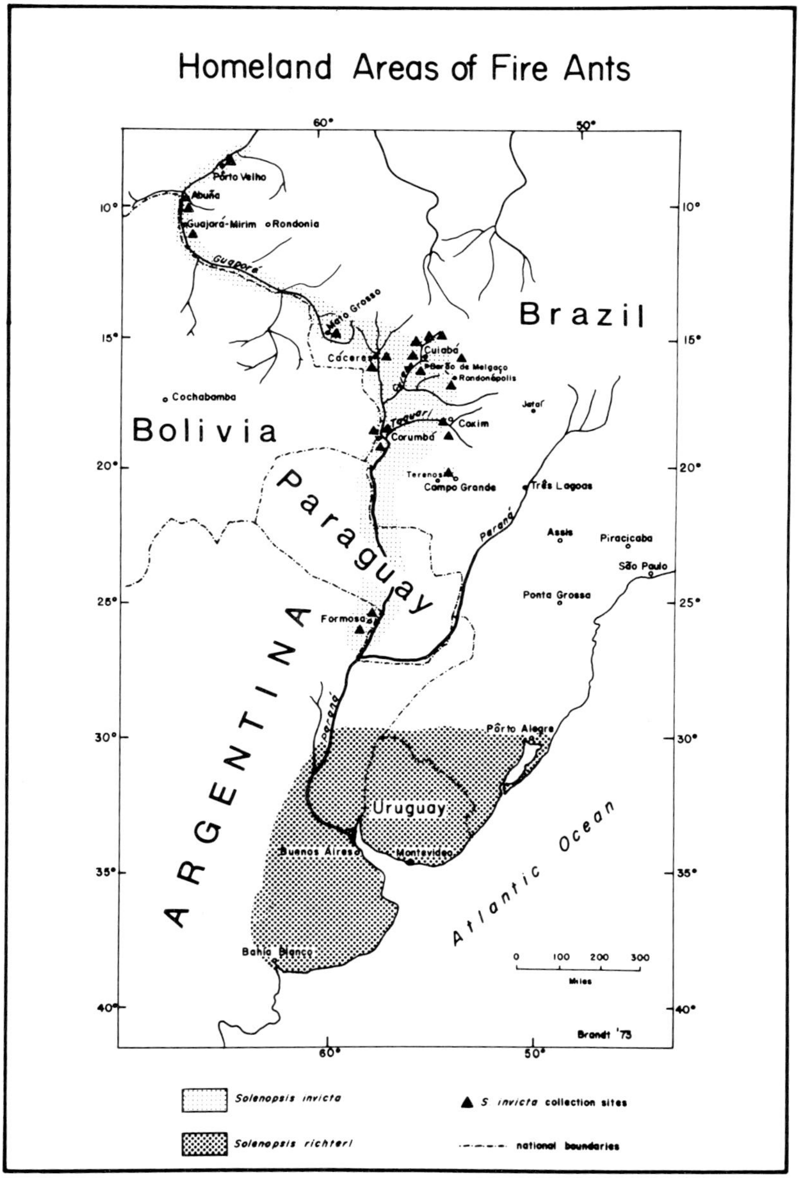

Figure 2. Distribution of *Solenopsis invicta* and *S. richteri* in South America.

Alabama, area sometime between 1933 and 1941. It has been extremely successful in the United States and now occupies major areas in North Carolina, South Carolina, Georgia, Florida, Alabama, Mississippi, Louisiana, Texas, and a small region in Arkansas. This ant is usually light reddish-brown, but it may range to a dark brown color. The mounds of *S. invicta* are more rounded than those of *S. richteri*.

Solenopsis xyloni McCook.—The southern fire ant is a native species. It has been largely displaced and eliminated in the southeastern United States by *S. invicta* but still exists in fringe areas. It is difficult to distinguish this species from *S. invicta* by color, but the two are usually separable by microscopic examination of morphologic characteristics. *S. xyloni* exists in smaller colonies than *S. invicta* and never builds an obvious rounded or conical mound. It is less aggressive, and its sting is much less severe with mild pain and rare pustule formation.

Solenopsis geminata Fabricius.—The tropical fire ant is often listed as native to the United States, but it probably is not. It is likely that the species originated in northern South America and Central America and was spread worldwide, including the West Indies and southern United States, in the sixteenth and seventeenth centuries by commerce. It has been largely displaced in the southern United States by *S. invicta* but still exists in large numbers of colonies in South Florida and in parts of Central Florida, where it appears to be resisting the advance of *S. invicta*. *S. geminata* occurs in two color phases, red and black. Mounds, except for very small ones, are not constructed. This ant is not as aggressive as and its sting is less painful than that of *S. invicta*.

Since its introduction, *S. richteri* has spread slowly and enjoyed some success. With the introduction of *S. invicta* in about 1940, *richteri* also has been displaced and has been successful in holding only a small area in northern Mississippi (7). *S. invicta* has thrived and now occupies over 127 million acres in 13 southeastern states (see Fig. 1) (11). The only factors which have limited spread have been the heavy winter kill conditions to the north, competition from *S. geminata* in South Florida, and the desert conditions of West Texas. The adaptability of *S. invicta* is quite impressive. It has been found successfully inhabiting areas with light winter frosts, and one colony was found in Florida on a sandbar that was covered by the tide twice a day (12). It does extremely well on disturbed land, such as roadsides and farmland. In its native environment of the Paraguay River basin, it must exist in the presence of annual flooding. The ants respond to this by clinging together and forming a ball. In doing so, they trap air and become sufficiently buoyant to float down the river to a new nesting site. They are frequently found setting up housekeeping on logs floating down the river. It is interesting that this ball is so buoyant and rotates enough so that few, if any, of the ants are drowned in the process (7).

The inherent aggressiveness and adaptability of *S. invicta* cannot entirely account for its extreme success in the United States. In its native Brazil, it occupies an apparently stable area, and it has not successfully invaded surrounding territories (see Fig. 2) (13). The exact mechanisms which control its territorial distribution are not clear but appear to be related both to climatic conditions and probably natural parasites and disease states, some of which are now being identified. This may partially explain how *S. richteri* holds what territory it does against *S. invicta*, since the environmental conditions of that area resemble closely the normal habitat of *S. richteri* (an area where *S. invicta* does not exist in South America). The success of *S. invicta* can better be understood when one considers how much man has altered the environment during the last century. The southern United States was primarily a forested area. Forests were stripped from large areas, the land was disturbed through farming and urban development, and a new environment was created. The native fauna of largely forest-dwelling ants was not terribly successful at taking advantage of this new environment. The imported fire ant was then introduced into an ecological vacuum and rapidly outcompeted most of the other occupants. *S. invicta* has done extremely well on this disturbed land, i.e., cultivated farmland, pastureland, roadsides, suburban yards, etc. Heavily infested farmland may have over 100 colonies per acre, and individual colonies may contain from 50,000 to 250,000 ants (14). Such land becomes less useful from the commercial standpoint since the grazing of animals is hindered and farm machinery, particularly mowers and harvesters, may be damaged when they strike the ant mounds.

A recent survey conducted in 261 counties in 6 southern states estimated that in 1972 the imported fire ant was responsible for a total loss of income to the farmer of $48 million in *these counties alone*; the estimated decrease in land values was $500 million (15). Other reports have estimated that up to 16 percent of the young of quail and other ground-nesting birds were killed each year by the imported fire ant in heavily infested areas (16).

Taxonomy

The relationship of the fire ant to other hymenoptera is shown in Table 1. The taxonomy of the imported fire ant has been confusing and has only recently been established by Dr. William Buren of the University of Florida (17).

Anatomy

The imported fire ant is a small-to-medium size ant (3–6 mm). It is neither large nor bright red as many believe, but it gets its name from the burning sting it produces. Its anatomy is typical of all ants: it has a rigid exoskeleton divided into three basic body regions—head, alitrunk, and gaster. The alitrunk and gaster are separated by a thin waist, petiole, and postpetiole (Figs. 3, 4). The locations of various exocrine glands are shown in Figure 5. The ant is unable to pass solid food through its gastrointestinal tract. It subsists entirely on liquids and is very effective at extracting them. I have seen fire ants convert a hard-boiled egg to a dry powder in a matter of hours. The ant also has a crop, which serves as a "social stomach" where liquids are stored before being carried back to the colony and regurgitated to the queen and nest workers. This is probably a key element in the evolution of a social structure since it allows work specialization, i.e., nursemaids, queen attendants, housekeepers, workers, and soldiers. These role determinations are quite clear-cut in some species of ants, although not highly developed in the fire ant group. Note the stinger (Fig. 4), which is a modified ovapositer with associated venom gland, at the tip of the abdomen. Some species of ants have nonfunctional stingers, and a large group has no stingers at all. Of those without stingers, many (subfamily Formicinae) produce formic acid, which acts as a poison or repellent that the ant is able to ejaculate as a spray.[2]

2. The stinging ants (subfamilies Myrmicinae, Ponerinae, and others) do not produce formic acid.

TABLE 1. Taxonomy of the Imported Fire Ant

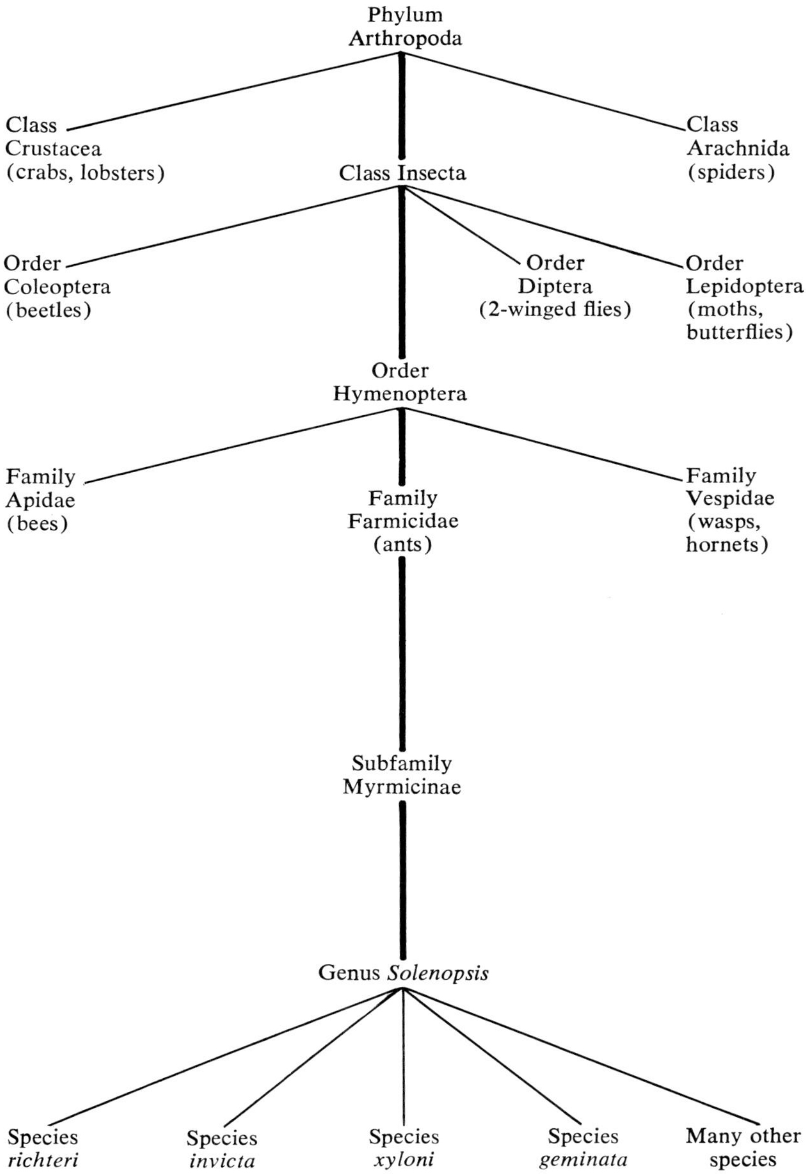

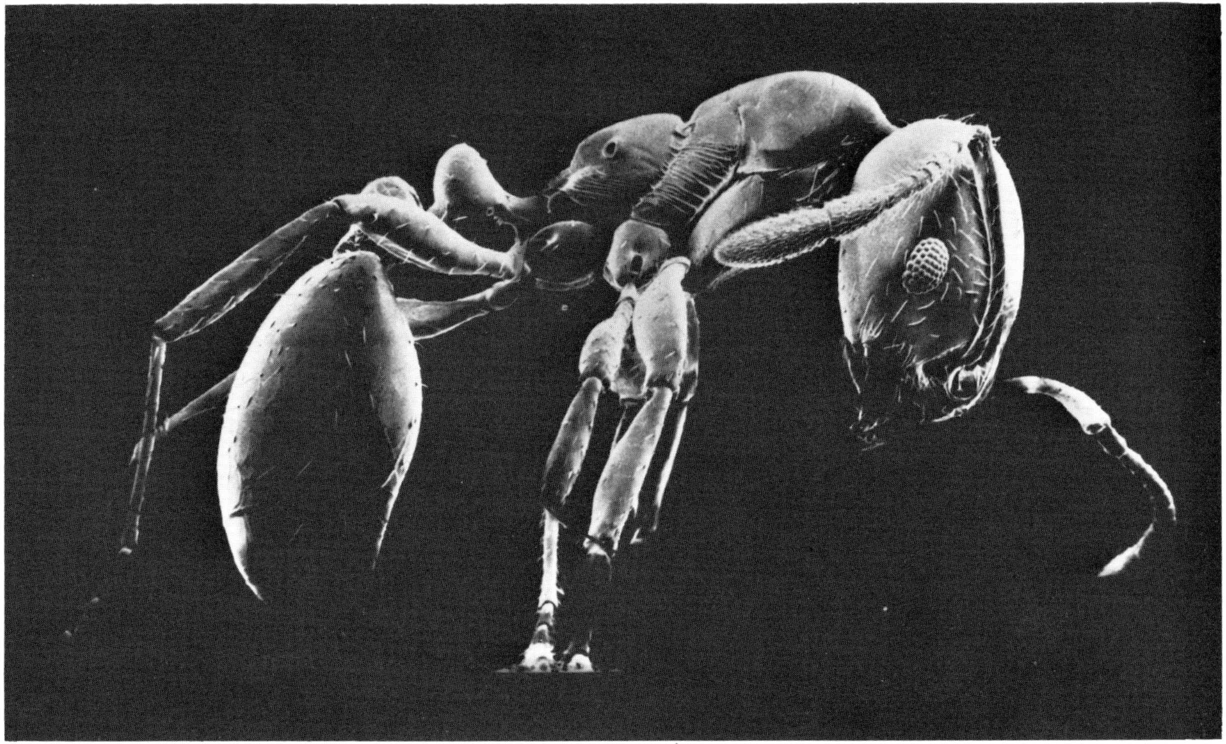

Figure 3. Scanning electron photomicrograph of imported fire ant worker. (Courtesy of USDA Section, University of Florida.)

LIFE CYCLE AND BEHAVIOR

The life cycle of the fire ant resembles in many ways that of the bee. After a colony is well established (usually more than 1 year old) (11), winged females (virgin queens) and winged males are produced. The queen and the alate sexuals are several times the size of the major workers. This marks one difference between the ants and the bees: the bee colony will tolerate only one queen at any given time, while fire ant colonies can be found with several thousand virgin queens and with even more than one functional queen in the same colony (11, 14, 18, 19). Control

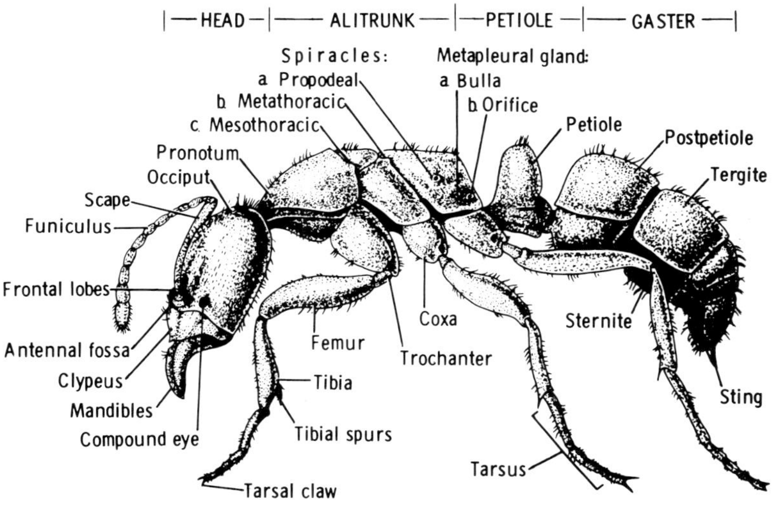

Figure 4. Ant anatomy. (Modified from Wilson [3].)

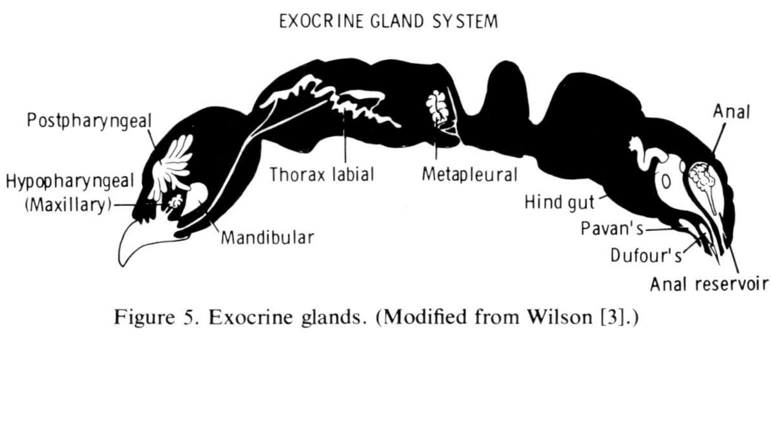

Figure 5. Exocrine glands. (Modified from Wilson [3].)

mechanisms of the mating behavior are unknown, but the most usual time for a mating flight is during the spring and early summer after a rain. Rhoades and Davis reported mating flights of *S. invicta* only when the relative humidity was over 80 percent and the temperature was 24–32°C (20). At some unknown stimulus, thousands of males fly up simultaneously from colonies over a large area and layer out at various altitudes of about 90–300 m. The male, who contributed nothing to the colony, now prepares to fulfill his only function (21).[3] Thirty to 60 minutes after the flight of the males, there is a spontaneous coordinated flight of virgin queens from many colonies in the area (22). They ascend into the swarm of males and mate quickly. In one brief blaze of glory, the males perform their function as sperm dispensers, following which they wander aimlessly and soon fall prey to predators. The queen mates in flight with several males, thereby obtaining her lifetime supply of sperm. These sperm remain viable for years, and although the lifetime of the queen is not documented, it is known to be at least in excess of 4 years for the imported fire ant and over 15 years for many other ants (7). (The life span of the queen termite may well be more than 30 years.) The magnitude of these nuptial flights is difficult to comprehend until one considers how easy it is to collect large numbers of queens for scientific study. All one has to do is to start with a heavily infested area such as the Tampa Bay area in Florida, pick a Sunday afternoon after a spring rain, and go to a shopping center parking lot. There hundreds of newly mated queens can be found wandering about the asphalt trying to dig nests. One need only pick them up (23).[4]

Upon landing, the now fertile queen digs into the ground, making an initial chamber (90 percent of the queens have completed their burrows within 6–7 hours) (19).[5] Before digging, she breaks off her wings and subsequently catabolizes the wing muscles as a source of energy. She generally begins laying eggs immediately. The *S. invicta* queen lays 15–20 eggs in 2–3 days. Glancy re-

3. Forbes observed that in preparation for the nuptial flight the males of *Camponotus americanus* void the gut and their abdomens fill with air, thus improving their aerodynamics (21).

4. After a major nuptial flight, as many as 6 queens per square yard have been found (45,000/acre) (23).

5. In heavily infested areas, 2–5 queens have been observed cooperatively setting up one nest (19).

ported 26–58 percent of the first eggs are trophic eggs, which are fed to the larvae. When the larvae hatch at 4–7 days, they rotate their heads until they find a trophic egg to eat. The time from the start of egg-laying until the first workers have eclosed from their cocoons is highly variable. The fire ant has generally produced some workers to help her within 24–30 days (14, 19). By 60 days, the queen has 85 workers, 1,000 at 5 months, 11,000 at 1 year, and 230,000 at 3 years (maturity) (14). A mature colony may then produce 2,300–4,500 new queens per season (23).[6]

Ants undergo complete metamorphosis as is characteristic of all higher (holometabolous) insects. During the larval stage, the young are fed by the worker ants. The larvae will enter the pupal stage and develop into the adult form without further nourishment. The life cycle of the fire ant serves as a fairly good model for most of the ants. Some of the more fascinating variations in mating pattern and life-style deserve further comment.

The "bulldog" ants of the genus *Myrmecia* were the subject of a pictorial essay in *National Geographic* (25). They hold great fascination for ant-watchers because they are one of the most primitive types of ant, have a rather low degree of socialization, and are among the largest of ant species, ranging up to 36 mm in length (3). They are aggressive and formidable, the stings being extremely painful and indeed dangerous. Moreover, they see quite well and can leap at an intruder. Within the colony, hunting is performed largely by individuals. The new queen leaves the nest intermittently to forage for prey, an arrangement which is termed partial claustration and is generally considered a primitive trait (Table 2).

An interesting variation in life cycle is seen in *Monomorium pharaonis*, the Pharaoh's ant (26). The nuptial flight no longer occurs, winged members are not produced, and new colonies are formed by a process called budding. *M. pharaonis* has become a specialist. Originally a native of Africa, it has spread throughout the world as a stowaway on ships and boats. Its association with man has been sealed by its adaptation to living in the cracks and crevices of man's dwellings, where it is a general pest. In adapting to this environment, however, Pharaoh's ant has done more than simply give up the mating flight. Although it would first

6. *Myrmica rubra* may have to wait 2 years for her first workers, during which time she remains sealed in her nest (24).

appear that budding simply involves the splitting off of a group of workers along with virgin queens and males, surprisingly it turned out that the budding of a group with such virgin queens, males, and workers would not result in another colony unless immature brood was also taken along. It was then even more surprising to

TABLE 2. BEHAVIORAL AND OTHER TRAITS OF *Myrmecia*

Primitive Traits

1. Multiple queens occur in many nests.
2. The eggs are spherical and lie apart from one another on the nest floor.
3. The larvae are fed directly with fresh insect fragments.
4. The larvae are able to crawl short distances unaided.
5. The adults are highly nectarivorous and collect insects mainly as food for the larvae.
6. Transport of one adult by another is rare, awkward in execution, and not accompanied by tonic immobility on the part of the transportee.
7. There is neither recruitment among workers to food sources nor any other apparent form of cooperation during foraging.
8. Alarm communication is slow and inefficient; the nature of the signal is still unknown.
9. Colony founding is only partially claustral.
10. When deprived of workers, nest queens can revert to colony-founding behavior, including foraging aboveground.

Advanced Traits (also found in higher ants)

1. The queen and sterile worker castes are very distinct from each other, and intermediates are rare.
2. Worker polymorphism occurs in many species, manifested as the coexistence of two well-defined worker subcastes.
3. The colonies are moderately large and the nests regular and fairly elaborate in construction.
4. Regurgitation occurs both among adults and from adults to larvae.
5. Adults groom each other as well as the brood.
6. Trophic eggs are laid by the workers and fed to other workers and the queen.
7. The workers cover the larvae with soil just prior to pupation, thus aiding them in spinning cocoons, and they assist the newly eclosed adults in emerging from the cocoons.
8. Nest odors exist, and territorial behavior among colonies is well developed.

SOURCE: Wilson (3).

find that the queens and males were not necessary to the new colony formation, and if a group of workers were given only young brood they would rear these individuals into queens and males which would then mate and establish a new colony (24). If a virgin queen were isolated with workers, her offspring would all be male until she was able to be fertilized.

There are three concepts here that are generally difficult to grasp. They apply, however, to *all* of the ants, the bees, and, in fact, to all the hymenoptera: all 250,000 or more members of one colony are first generation offspring of one queen; all but a few members of the colony are *female* (daughters of the queen); and males are haploid, the product of unfertilized eggs, while females are diploid, a rather alien concept to those of us accustomed to mammalian genetics. To conceptualize in mammalian standards, the male ant is a "clone of sperm cells." The fascination of this is increased even further when one considers that in honeybees the queen of this so-called lower life form can voluntarily elect whether or not to fertilize one given egg from within her spermotheca via a voluntary sphincter. Moreover, her election to fertilize or not is determined by the cell presented to her by the workers. Drone cells are somewhat larger than worker cells, and the queen will therefore deposit an unfertilized egg in the larger cell, or a fertilized egg in the smaller cell.

The mechanisms of fertilization in sex determination and queen determination in the bee (*Apis mellifera*) have been well studied. The similar control mechanisms for the ants are essentially unknown, with the exception of the findings of one experiment regarding queen determination, which will be discussed later. It is clear, however, that the winged male and female, particularly the male, are generally produced after the colony is mature, well established, and has a large force of workers (14).

One of the most interesting of all the ant adaptations is that of the Myrmicine tribe, Attini. Comprising 11 genera and 200 species, it has been immensely successful in Central and South America. These are the leaf cutter, or parasol, ants, so-called because they carry pieces of leaves over their heads, thus resembling a parasol. An enjoyable historical account is given by Von Hagen (27):

> My Indian servants, dusky, kinky-haired Miskito men, lamented all this work. It was useless, quoth a toothless elder, to plant anything but bananas or manioc, as the Wiwis were sure to cut off all the leaves. Without the slightest encouragement the Miskito Indians would launch forth on the tales of the ravages of the "Wiwi Laca," but unswayed by the illustrations, like Pangloss I could only remark that

> all this was very well but let us cultivate our garden. In two weeks the carrots, the cabbages, the turnips were doing well. The carrots had unfurled their fernlike tops, the cabbage grew as if by magic. From our small palm-thatched house my wife and I cast admiring eyes over our jungle garden. Our mind called forth dishes of steaming vegetables to replace dehydrated greens and the inevitable beans and yucca. Even the toothless elder came by and admitted that white man's energy had overcome the lethargy of the Indian. Then the catastrophe fell upon us. We arose one morning and found our garden defoliated: every cabbage leaf was stripped, the naked stem was the only thing above the ground. Of the carrots nothing was seen. In the center of the garden, rising a foot in height, was a conical peak of earth, and about it were dry bits of earth, freshly excavated. Into a hole in the mound, ants, moving in quickened step, were carrying bits of our cabbage, tops of the carrots, the beans—in fact our entire garden was going down that hole. I could see the grinning face of the toothless Miskito Indian. The Wiwis had come.

The elegant specialization of the *Atta* species is that they have become fungus farmers and have developed a truly symbiotic relationship with a particular fungus of the Basidiomycetes group. The *Atta* workers forage for fresh vegetation. They bring the leaves back to the nest where they cut them into 1–2 mm pieces, chew and macerate the edges of these pieces, add salivary secretions until the leaves are wet and pulpy, and then add a drop of anal fluid to the leaf. They then pluck mycelia from other parts of the fungus garden and plant several of them on the prepared substratum. In trying to discover the mechanism by which the ants could maintain a pure culture of this fungus (since unattended nests were quickly overgrown with contaminant fungi), Martin et al. (28) looked for fungustatic activity in the secretions of the ant. Much to their amazement they discovered another piece of the puzzle. Not only are the anal secretions not fungustatic but they facilitate the fungus growth. As it turns out, the fungus lacks the ability to digest protein, thus severely limiting its chances for survival. The fecal fluid from the ant contains all the amino acids necessary to accelerate growth of the fungus, so the fungus can take full advantage of its cellulose-digesting capabilities, returning the cellulose to the ant amply in the form of gonglydia. The term gonglydia was coined by Wheeler to describe small buds from the hyphae of the fungus. These swellings at the ends of the hyphae are 30–50 μ in diameter and are the ants' only food. They do not eat the hyphae. The fungus has been pruned of its sexual phase for so long that even when grown in culture it will not fully develop a sexual phase and therefore is an unclassifiable fungus. It has no need for a sexual phase since the ant guarantees its existence. When establishing a new colony, the *Atta* queen fills her buccal pouch with mycelia and carries these to the new nest location on her nuptial flight. Her first act upon digging her nest is to spit out this wad of hyphae and set up the fungus garden, even before she begins to lay eggs. During this period, the queen does not eat any of the fungus garden but rather eats some of her own eggs for sustenance. These special eggs, found in almost all ant species, are called trophic eggs, or "omelets." They are ill-formed eggs that are fused in groups of two or more and are apparently produced to be eaten.

The discovery that the anal secretions were nutrient medium in no way clarified the mystery of the ant's ability to maintain a pure culture. It remained for Weber in 1957 (29) to complete the puzzle by careful observation of the amazing fact that these ants actually weed their garden. The ant recognizes early growth of an alien fungus and carefully destroys the foreign hyphae with its mandibles, then grooms and cleans itself.

Martin et al. (28) calculated that one colony of *Atta columbica* contained between 1 and 2.5 million workers. Respect for these creatures increases even further with the observation that a crude ventilation system exists in the *Atta* nest (30). Smoke introduced at peripheral openings in the nest rises from the central openings. This is caused by the convection current produced by the high rate of metabolism and decay in the area of the fungus gardens near the center of the colony.

Another fascinating mutualistic relationship exists between a group of plants called myrmecophytes and the ants which inhabit them. It is almost as though a contract had been drawn up between the two.The tree's contribution to the union is housing in the form of hollow or soft, pithy, easily excavated cavities of thorns or branches, which seem particularly suited to the ant colony. In addition, the tree has some unusual structures, such as "Mullerian bodies or detachable corpuscles called Beltian bodies on their leaflets'' (3). These structures are rich sources of nutrients and seem to have no discernible function or value to the tree, with the exception of attracting the ants. The advantage to the tree was a little less obvious until a study by Janzen (31) showed that the ant tenants protect the tree. He reported that if he destroyed the resident ant population in the bull's horn acacia, the unprotected trees suffered severe damage from insect pests, browsing mammals, and overgrowth by other plants.

A description of ant specialists would not be complete without the infamous and much misunderstood army and legionary ants. This broad grouping includes the genus *Eciton* (army ants) of South America and the genus *Anomma* of Africa (driver ants). Wheeler described the driver and legionary ants as the ''Huns and Tartars of the insect world'' (32). *Eciton* has been well studied. These ants were also the subject of a very popular movie quite a few years ago in which they ate up everything except Charlton Heston.[7] They really do not deserve their bad press (unless you happen to be an insect). The army ants are blind, but their other methods of communication are so well developed that this does not represent a significant handicap. Some 150,000–700,000 workers swarm forward at a steady pace, bringing down everything that cannot run away from them.[8] These ants do not build nests; instead, they form a mass of interlocking bodies over and around the queen and the brood. They will even link themselves together to form a living bridge over small chasms.

The queen is a truly prolific egg-layer. She can lay between 100,000 and 300,000 eggs within 2 weeks and has a massively swollen abdomen which is almost twice as large as the rest of her body. Again, we see an adaptation of mating behavior which is not quite as novel as that of the Pharaoh's ant but is more intermediate and in some ways resembles the behavior of the bees. Schneirla (33) studied this behavior extensively. He noted that at a particular point in time sexual members consisting of about 6 new queens and 1,500 males are produced. The workers begin to affiliate either with the mother queen or with the new alate sexuals. Then the two groups split. The new queens are

7. A historical note is supplied by Buren (7): Eleanor Parker was also spared, and close-ups in the film revealed members of *Pogonomyrmex* spp. and even a *Solenopsis* sp., but no army ants.

8. A colony of *Anomma* may number 22 million (7).

fertilized by males flying from other colonies, but the queens do not fly and remain within the colony. Only one queen is allowed to go off with the new bivouac. The rest of the daughter queens and the males are "sealed off" by the workers, held behind, and eventually pushed aside and left to die. At that point there are two colonies, but without any winged males or excess females.

Role Specialization

A key element in the life of the ant which sets it apart from most of the other insects is that of caste and role determination. It is this ability to specialize in roles and the social structure that goes with it which has allowed the great success of the ants. Our model, the imported fire ant, has been studied extensively by Wilson (4). In some species there is a good correlation between body size and work role. In the case of the fire ants, however, there is an overlapping bimodal size frequency distribution of roughly two different size classes of workers within the colony. A sampling of the workers at various tasks showed no relationship between size and work task, although there was a slightly higher proportion of larger workers foraging outside the nest (4). "In these species (*S. geminata*), therefore, we see a moderate degree of polymorphism (size variation) associated with a relatively weak degree of polyethism (division of labor)" (4). In *Formica obscuripes*, the worker caste is weakly polymorphic yet strongly polyethic with the larger individuals remaining in the nest while the smaller ones do most of the foraging. Other species exist in which there are both marked differences in size and configuration and rigid role assignments associated with the different sized classes. Large workers of the African weaver ant (*Oecophylla longinoda*) do most of the foraging and nest construction, while the smaller workers remain in and around the nest, caring for the brood and queen and keeping the nest clean. The extreme of role assignment is seen in some species of *Myrmecocystus* and *Melophorus*, in which certain young members of the largest class are transformed into "honey pots." This is another example of a common theme throughout the ant society: the sacrifice of one for the good of the colony. In this case, the ant's general inability to store a food reserve is answered by a specific role assignment. A young major worker is by some method selected and then grossly overfed by the foraging workers with nectar or honeydew transported and regurgitated from their social stomachs. This young worker generally attaches itself to the ceiling and is fed continually until it is swollen. In this gorged state it is basically unable to move but is an emergency food reserve for the rest of the colony, who will drain the "honey pot" when the colony's survival is threatened by the loss of available food sources.

One of the important role specializations is the development of the soldier caste. Their anatomy is adapted in a way which is very suitable to their task as defenders of the colony. Their body size and jaws are generally more massive than those of the worker, and their heads are large and bulky. Wheeler (34) pointed out that the change in head configuration is largely accounted for by enlargement of the adductor muscles of the mandibles, which greatly supplements the shearing and crushing power of the jaws. In addition, the mandibles in some species are pointed or hook-shaped, augmenting their piercing ability (most noted in the army ants *Eciton* and *Anomma*). Army ant soldiers line up along the flanks of the columns with their heads facing outward and upward, jaws open (3).

The anatomic modification of the head into a shield shape in some species presents a smooth armor-plated surface which can plug nest openings (35). During routine activity the soldiers appear sluggish and nonfunctional. They do not contribute to nest cleaning, brood tending, foraging, or any useful work. Their true function is not evident until an intruder (such as a member of another ant species) is introduced into the nest, at which time they quickly become aroused and rush toward it. If the trespasser is attacking, the soldiers will quickly block the nest openings with their heads, jaws gaping. They will then attempt to grasp the intruder's mandibles and crush them, thus putting it out of action. As the strength of the attack diminishes, the soldiers will emerge from the nest and engage the enemy, generally coming up from its rear and attempting to cut it in half at the waist, putting it out of action in a short while. The attack is thus a highly organized one: first defense, then offense with all attack sequences intended either to put the enemy out of commission or to kill it quickly, rather than randomly chopping off antennae or parts of legs. This specialization is made even more impressive by the behavior of certain soldiers (i.e., *Camponotus* spp.) which serve as living gates (3). The nest openings are so constructed that they can be blocked by the head of the soldier which then presents to the outside only a flat shield and open jaws. This position is maintained until a returning worker approaches the opening and is identified, at which time the soldier backs off and allows the worker to enter. The soldier then returns to its post.

Another fascinating example of role specialization and cooperation is exhibited by the fungus-growing ant *Atta cephalotes*. The major workers forage and return to the nest with a large piece of leaf in their jaws; thus, fully occupied, they are vulnerable to a natural enemy, a parasitic phorid fly (36). This problem is resolved by having one of the small workers ride on the apex of the piece of leaf which the major worker is carrying over its head. This small worker's contribution seems to be to watch for the approach of the phorid fly and to repel it by fencing with its jaws and hind legs, thus protecting the major worker from attack. With this sort of exquisite specialization and cooperation, it soon becomes clear why the ants have enjoyed such success.

The most critical role adaptation of all is that of the queen. There are very limited data about the mechanism of queen determination, and the genetics are difficult to grasp for those with a background in mammalian genetics. It is quite possible for the queen and many of her worker daughters within a colony to have the identical genome. In spite of this, there are extreme differences in size, behavior, hormonal function, pheromone production, and behavior between the worker and the queen. If ovarian plates are taken from the developing worker and transplanted into a developing queen larvae, the ovaries become functional. The mechanism of queen determination in the honeybee is well understood and is referred to early in this book. In the bees, the queen is clearly determined by the addition of large amounts of nutrient-rich royal jelly to any female larvae. This has not been well demonstrated in the ant. In one control mechanism, it has been shown that in certain species in the presence of a viable queen, many of the larger larvae are repeatedly bitten or stung by the workers, resulting in runting. It has been suggested that female ant larvae are determined as queens with the aid of a special protein-rich diet, the analogue of royal jelly (3).

2
SENSES AND COMMUNICATION

The sensory capabilities of the ant are indeed incredible, considering its level of evolution and its physical dimensions.

Vision

Since a great deal more research has been done on the honeybee than on the ant, some general information regarding its vision will be mentioned first, and this data will then be compared with that of the fire ant and other ants. The basic unit of vision in the bee and the ant is the rhadomore. This is a collection of 8 highly modified, spindle-shaped nerve cells which terminate in retinal nerve fibers. Each of these visual units is in direct proximity to its concave lens with no separation equivalent to the aqueous and vitreous humors of the human eye. Thus, there is no equivalent of the image-focusing lens and high sensitivity of the human fovia. Instead, each unit transmits its own image, resulting in a compound picture. In the honeybee, there are approximately 6,300 lens-rhadomore units (ommatidia) per eye, each giving overlapping images. On the basis of training experiments, it has been established that the honeybee is able to distinguish two points which subtend an angle of approximately 1°. This compares with the visual discrimination of the human eye of an arc subtending .01°. The bee's visual field is fuzzy; it perceives only vague images yet is able to see in almost all directions around its body simultaneously and is exquisitely sensitive to movement. The amount of light required for the bee to see an image is approximately the same as for man. The color vision range is shifted from that which we are accustomed to in that its sensitivity starts in the ultraviolet range and ends in the yellow or near red range. This ultraviolet vision allows it to see the sun on overcast days and to see on flowers ultraviolet markings which are totally invisible to us. Both the bee and ant can evaluate the plane of polarized sunlight (37, 38). Therefore, they can orient and find the way home or to a food supply simply by being allowed to see a patch of blue sky.

The vision of the fire ant is fairly comparable to that of the honeybee (3). The optic lobes of the army ant degenerate while still in the pupal stage, and it has no eyes as is the case in certain subterranean genera (i.e., *Carebara*). At the other extreme, certain of the arboreal species have thousands of ommatidia per eye. A visual acuity greater than that of the honeybee has been demonstrated in *Formica rufa* (39, 40). The visual spectrum of the fire ant ranges from below 350 mμ in the near ultraviolet range to 650 mμ in the orange, with a peak sensitivity at 350, 505, and 620 mμ (41). Fire ants and other species (*Formica rufa*) respond in a predictable manner to certain visual patterns. They prefer closed to open figures and prefer white areas on black with vertical black-white borders.

Another interesting aspect of the visual capacities of the ants and bees is that of sun compass orientation. This phenomenon in ants was discovered by Felix Santschi in 1911 when he tried to determine how desert ants could return directly to their nests over shifting sands. He was able to show by the use of mirrors that if the apparent position of the sun were shifted to the opposite side, the ant would reverse his direction 180° and proceed in a straight line away from the nest. This was well demonstrated in the case of the fire ant by Marak and Wolken (41), who placed food on a table illuminated by a single light source. Upon finding this, the fire ant would return directly to its nest. If on this return trip the light was switched off and another light on the opposite side of the table switched on, the ant would reverse its direction 180°. By first turning on one light, then the other, it is possible to get the fire ant to march back and forth like a robot. Wilson (42) has shown that individual fire ants may initially follow an odor trail from the nest but will eventually forage on their own. When foraging alone, they orient visually, and while returning they will lay down an odor trail which will be followed by the recruited workers to the new food source.

One's respect for this sun compass orientation is further increased when considering the fact that in foraging, the ant or the bee will generally wander from one direction to another in an irregular zigzag manner until it encounters a food source. It then returns to the nest, using its sun compass, by the shortest possible route, the so-called beeline. In order to accomplish this feat, the ant or bee must do the equivalent of integral calculus (or at least triangulation) to take into account the angle of deviation and the magnitude of his meanderings off of the beeline during his foraging activity. In addition, it has been shown that the bee (43) or the ant (*Formica rufa*) (44) is also computing the movement of the sun during the time period that it is out foraging, perhaps several hours. Although it is intuitively obvious that if this fact were not taken into account there would be a time-related error in the return flight, it was not until Jander's experiment (44) that this was proven to be so. In the bee, this error can be introduced by placing the returning worker bee in the dark for several hours and subsequently releasing it, resulting in an error in its return flight commensurate with the sun's movement of 15° of arc per hour times the amount of time the worker was kept in the dark. This same phenomenon was experimentally demonstrated in ants (43). In addition to all these capabilities, it has also been demonstrated that the ant can make the same return trip if the image of the sun is blocked out and it is given only a patch of blue sky with which to orient (39). It has been shown that the ant makes use of the pattern of polarized light to calculate the sun's position.

HEARING

The ant is basically deaf to airborne sound but is highly sensitive to ground vibrations which it perceives through sensors on the leg. Sound generated by the ant, presumably for communication purposes, is produced by a process called stridulation, that is, the rubbing together of special body parts to produce a chirp exactly as the cricket does. In a number of ant subfamilies this sound is in the audible range of the human ear. For instance, *Pogonomyrmex occidentalis* produces a low energy 1–4 kc per second note on the downstroke and a louder or higher energy 7–9 kc per second note on the return stroke, and the sound is heard as a faint continuous squeak (3). The frequency range produced by *Solenopsis* is well above the human spectrum. It has recently been recorded with electronic equipment and is well above the audible range (12). The function of stridulation has been confusing. In my own observations of fire ant colonies, and those of others with much more experience, stridulation seems to occur at random times, frequently when the colony is undisturbed. In addition, stridulation produced no apparent response in surrounding ants. However, there is evidence in certain species (i.e., *Pogonomyrmex* spp. and some of the leaf-cutting ants) that when a worker is trapped it will begin stridulating, and stridulation of a trapped worker in a cave-in results in recruitment of other workers, who rapidly begin digging the trapped worker out. Thus, stridulation may serve as an underground alarm system in the case of a cave-in.[1]

Touch

Wilson does not feel that tactile stimuli have a significant role in communication (3). One certainly observes a phenomenon which has been called antennal language. From my own observations, this occurs frequently and is often seen when one worker is returning from a food find and encounters another worker. They will come together and apparently tap antennae for a few seconds. After this encounter, the contacted ant may follow the trail of the returning ant back to the food source. It is Wilson's feeling, however, that during the antennation, there is probably sampling of chemical stimuli on the body surface of the ant rather than actual communication through the antennae tapping.

Taste

The sense of taste has been investigated in both the bees and the ants (3). The hymenoptera "taste" by contact with chemoreceptors in the antennae. Strangely enough, they are relatively insensi-

1. Although bees also perceive sound through their legs, an interesting application of sound communication has been observed. As an established colony prepares to swarm with the old queen leaving the nest to set up a new one, several larvae are fed royal jelly and develop into queens. The first young queen to emerge produces an audible sound called piping or tooting. The enclosed queens which have not emerged respond with a lower frequency note called quacking. The duet continues for days until the first emerged queen has left with another group of workers (after swarm) at which time one of the enclosed queens emerges. Since bee colonies will tolerate only one queen at a time, this apparent sound communication would seem to eliminate the need for mortal combat between a number of young queens emerging simultaneously. Both of these notes are clearly audible to the human ear.

tive to the recognition of sweet substances. In addition, they fail to react to a number of the hexoses and the pentoses which we perceive as sweet. Also, several species of ants are more sensitive than the bees or man to certain of the disaccharides and trisaccharides. Taste does not seem to be a major sense.

Time

It has been well demonstrated that honeybee workers can be taught to return to the food source at the same time each day by a training procedure similar to that used by Pavlov. A similar ability has been demonstrated in certain species of ants (i.e., *Formica rufa*). Once again, one's respect mounts for this creature who can correct for the movement of the sun over time and who also can be trained to tell time in seeking a reward.

Smell

The sense of smell is remarkably developed in the ant. Certainly, it far outclasses the abilities of smell in man. The organs responsible for taste and smell are the antennae. In the honeybee, at least nine different types of sensory organs have been identified on the antennae, making them more sophisticated than the identifiable sensory organelles of human skin. A bee can be taught new odors more quickly and retain the memory longer than any other kind of stimulus, including visual (3). The olfactory threshold for a wide number of compounds has been worked out for the ants, bees, and man, and is almost identical in all three with the maximal sensitivity in the ant. The threshold of the ant *Acanthomyops claviger* is lowest for the C_{11} compound of an alkene series and requires a concentration between 10^{11} and 10^{12} molecules per cubic centimeter for detection (45). The ant again surpasses man's capabilities in its capacity to "smell" a CO_2 gradient in trace amounts. According to Wilson (42), fire ant workers will tend to move up a CO_2 gradient and thus in the direction of the largest nearby cluster of ants digging through barriers placed in their way. Thus, CO_2 is the simplest pheromone. In addition, it has been demonstrated that the fire ant can detect and move up a vapor gradient.

The sense of smell also apparently plays a significant role in housekeeping within the colony. The social insects are quite fastidious in their habits, keeping the inside of their nests meticulously clean and carefully walling off immovable "foreign bodies" within the nest. They also constantly groom and clean themselves and each other. Depending on the species, dead ants are either eaten or carried off and discarded, generally in one location, producing a sort of burial mound. It has been shown in *Solenopsis*, as well as in *Pogonomyrmex badius*, that a worker upon contacting a recently deceased or immobilized nestmate will groom it in the normal way. If the body is allowed to decompose in the open air for a day or so, the worker will investigate briefly with antennae then pick up the deceased and carry it away to the refuse pile. Paper treated with acetone extracts of such corpses receives the same treatment (3). Such extracts have implicated long chain fatty acids and their esters. Oleic acid serves this purpose well, and this compound has been identified in the corpses of *Solenopsis* (46). The narrow-minded, stereotyped nature of this response is demonstrated by the painting of live nestmates with oleic acid. These live ants, marked with the chemical, are picked up unprotesting and carted off to the refuse pile. If they then return to the nest without cleaning themselves adequately, they are treated as corpses and carted off to the refuse pile over and over again until the chemical odor has dissipated.

This behavior is made even more interesting by the fact that injured *Solenopsis* workers tend to leave the nest more readily when it is disturbed, and in some species (i.e., *Formica rufa*) workers fatally infected with a fungus will leave the nest and cling to blades of grass with their mandibles and legs just before dying. This behavior irresistibly raises the image of the old elephant going off to the sacred burial ground, and one must be reminded that these are only stereotyped behaviors of a primitive nervous system. Wilson (3), who has considerable experience with *Solenopsis*, comments that unlike most other ant genera, these ants consume a large part of their dead, at least under laboratory conditions. However, in my limited observation, even dismembered workers from other colonies of *S. invicta* are not cannibalized but are carted off whole and placed in a pile.

PHEROMONES

The sense of smell in communication is most widely applied in the area of pheromones. Pheromones are simple organic chemical compounds detected by chemoreceptors in the antennae—

"signals" which evoke certain behavior. Wilson (42) estimated that "almost the entire social organization of the fire ant might be mediated by as few as ten pheromones." By combining these simple compounds in various ratios, a wide variety of information can be transferred. The economy of this system has been worked out for the honeybee, where queen substance (identified as *trans*-9-keto-2-decenoic acid) is used to inhibit ovarial development in workers, to inhibit royal cell building by workers, and to attract workers during swarming. It also serves as a long-distance sex attractant and aphrodisiac, inducing copulation by males who reach the queen in flight (42). Another example is

TABLE 3. PHEROMONES OF *Solenopsis*

Chemical Stimulus (Pheromone)	Response
Co_2	Clustering and digging (41)
Queen-tending	Grooming and feeding of queen (49)
Brood-tending	Feeding and caring for brood (9)
Trail	Excitement following behavior (9, 41)
Alarm (trail and cephalic)	Excitement and orientation (controversial) (42)
Sex	Attraction and mating (presumed, but not proven)
Colony odor	Scanning and acceptance or rejection of introduced ant (presumed on behavioral grounds, but not proven)

isoamyl acetate, an alarm signal in the honeybee. Whenever one is stung by a honeybee, the stinger remains embedded in the victim, and part of the bee's abdomen is torn off, releasing isoamyl acetate, which attracts other bees to the attack. The same response can be achieved for the most part with isoamyl acetate alone.

Pheromones are generally in the C_7 to C_{20} range of relatively simple aliphatic compounds. Specific signals may vary only in the configuration around a double bond or in the relative proportions in which the chemicals are present. The antennal sensors are capable not only of detecting a *cis* from a *trans* isomer, but of doing so in picomolar amounts. They are also capable of integrating the information from both antennae in order to orient towards the source of these chemical emissions. The known pheromones of *Solenopsis* spp. are summarized in Table 3.

Trail pheromone.—One of the major developments in ant communication has been the development of the trail pheromone, which probably evolved from a more primitive form of communication—tandem walking or tandem calling. This is seen in more primitive genera (i.e., *Leptothorax muscorum*) and represents the transitional state between solitary hunting and the highly integrated foraging of the army ants, which is largely dependent on trail pheromone. Tandem running is characterized by a stereotyped motor display of invitational behavior during which an ant returning from a food find first approaches a nestmate and then regurgitates some of the newly found food to her. It then raises its gaster, exposing the stinger, and secretes a drop of venom. Nestmates are attracted by this poison gland substance (47).

Filter paper dummies impregnated with various chemicals were used to replace the calling ant. Stereotyped following behavior was seen only with pure poison substance or combinations containing poison gland substance. No response was seen with Dufour's gland substance or with scentless dummies. Nestmates respond to this poison gland secretion by approaching the caller. As soon as the caller is contacted on the hind legs by a follower, it runs forward a short distance, stops, and resumes the calling posture until the follower catches up and makes contact again. The procedure is then repeated. The leader then returns to the food source by visual orientation and without laying a chemical trail. This method is relatively inefficient, recruiting only one or two followers, and is time-consuming. An intermediate stage is found in *Camponotus* spp. where the leader, after recruiting a follower, no longer waits for the follower to catch up. Instead, it lays a short-lived odor trail which can be followed by as many as 10–20 workers.

The fire ant has a highly developed trail pheromone. Wilson and others have shown quite clearly that trailing behavior can be induced in *Solenopsis* spp. with artificial trails made from extracts of the fire ant's Dufour's gland (see Fig. 5). In fact, if a sufficiently strong trail is laid in a circular pattern, the fire ants will continue following it until they literally drop dead. The fire ant does not lay a trail while scouting, but does so upon returning from finding a new food source or nesting site. The recruited nestmates then follow the trail back to the food source, reinforcing the trail on their return. The army ants, on the other hand, lay scouting trails as well since they are unable to orient visually. Gas chromatographic examination of the fire ant trail substance indicates that it is a C_{16} to C_{17} compound (12). Wilson (3) estimates that each worker contains only a fraction of a nanogram (billionth of a gram). As the fire ant worker returns from a food source, it proceeds in a direct line using sun compass orientation; it proceeds deliberately, dragging its stinger along the ground and laying down minute droplets from its Dufour's gland. The workers in the nest respond by following the freshly laid trail back to the food source. Although they proceed in a straight line along the trail with considerable speed, they do not lay a pheromone trail of their own until evaluating and returning from the food source. Thus, the number of workers going to the food source builds up exponentially until the source is saturated, at which time disappointed workers return without laying a trail, and the magnitude of the stimulus gradually decreases as the food source decreases. This provides a type of qualitative control to an otherwise all-or-none phenomenon. As the recruited worker proceeds along the trail, it sweeps its antennae through the air, never touching the liquid trail itself, but analyzing the vapor cone given off by the liquid. By integrating the signal from both antennae simultaneously, the ant is able to move up the gradient of molecular concentration and orient on the trail with very little error. If the antennae are crossed or glued together, the ant becomes disoriented and follows the trail only with great difficulty (48). It would appear that towards the end of the trail the ant orients visually to its prey, allowing it to correct for movement of the prey from the original point of discovery and attack.

Specificity of the trail pheromones was determined by Wilson (42), who indicated that they are genera-specific and probably relate to the evolutionary closeness of the groups within the genus. *S. invicta* will follow an *S. xyloni* trail, but not that of the more distantly related *S. geminata*, whereas *geminata* will follow *xyloni* trails. *Solenopsis* trails, however, are never followed by other genera.

Although the trail communication of the honeybee, namely, the waggle dance, has been discussed earlier, it is helpful to briefly summarize it for comparison. A number of investigators have shown that a worker bee returning from a new food source will recruit sister bees by performing a stereotyped waggle dance. If performed at the entrance to the hive on a horizontal surface, it is executed in relationship to the sun. If done in the center of the hive, it is performed in the vertical plane with the line of gravity substituting for the sun. The bee vibrates its abdomen back and forth while running in a straight line, then returns in a circular manner to the point of origin and repeats the maneuver. The following information is transmitted in that manner: the angle of deviation from the sun to the food source is indicated by the angle of deviation between the long axis of the straight run from the sun; information concerning whether the deviation angle is to the right or the left of the sun is determined by the initial direction of movement of the tail as it starts to vibrate; and the distance to the food source is determined by the length of the straight run. Additional information regarding the nature of the food source is probably obtained by the sampling of chemicals and pollens carried on the worker's body. Thus, the bees tend to pollenate the same type of flower until the source is exhausted.

Although such a symbolic communication has not been shown in the ant, it is able to transfer the same amount of information by means of the trail pheromone. The manner in which it is laid down gives some information about distance and clearly gives direction with an even higher degree of resolution than the bee. Information about the nature of the food source can also be transmitted by food regurgitation and by examining the scout's body with the antennae. In a tropical rain forest where there are many obstacles to straight flight, bees use a chemical trail for recruitment by pausing at various sites along the return path to leave chemical markers, generally from the salivary glands. The trail is followed back by sister bees (i.e., *Trigona postica*) (49).

Queen-tending pheromone.—This pheromone causes workers to cluster about, groom, and feed the queen. Honeybee queen substance is *trans*-9-keto-2-decenoic acid, and its effectiveness is augmented by the addition of certain other compounds. Work with the fire ant queen-tending pheromone to date would suggest that it is also a combination. Extracts from queens reveal several fractions which produce queen-tending behavior. This effect is enhanced considerably by recombining these fractions (50). In addition, there seems to be some specificity to the mixtures since the maximal effect is on offspring of that queen as opposed to offspring of an unrelated queen.

Brood-tending pheromone.—In the case of the fire ant, the brood-tending pheromone has tentatively been identified as triolein, an 18-carbon triglyceride ester. This is produced by the immature forms (i.e., the brood) and elicits brood-tending behavior from the workers (12).

Alarm pheromone.—Wilson interpreted his observations of the alarmed *S. invicta* worker as an indication that there were simultaneous discharges of an alarm substance from the head and one or more trail substances from the Dufour's gland of the abdomen. The alarm substance alone would excite the workers without orienting, while the trail substance would orient without excitement. These two elements in combination resulted in orientation and alarm (51). Such a system is certainly theoretically satisfying. Attempts to reproduce this work, however, have been unsuccessful, and it is now doubtful that actual alarm pheromone is produced in the head of *Solenopsis* (7). Recently, Wilson has documented the use of a trail odor for alarm recruitment. Minor workers of *Pheidole dentata* when exposed to an intruder of certain species will go rapidly to the nest, laying down a trail from their poison gland. Rather than recruiting minor workers to return to a food source, soldiers are recruited to repel the attack (5). Interestingly, it is also specific in that the response is elicited primarily by the introduction of fire ants (the greatest threat to the colony). Other species of intruders are attacked by minor workers at the site without alarm recruitment of the soldiers. There are certainly some well-worked-out alarm pheromones, including the isoamyl acetate of the honeybee, formic acid of *Formica* spp., 4-methyl-3-heptanone of *Pogonomyrmex* spp., citronellal of *Acanthomyops claviger*, etc. (Fig. 6).

Alarm pheromones of the social insects fulfill certain logical criteria. First, they lie in the 5–10 carbon aliphatic hydrocarbon series with molecular weights between 100 and 200. Second, they are not species-specific (as one might expect from smaller weight compounds); in fact, they can be highly nonspecific, thus serving as general alarm substances. As indicated previously, the maximal sensitivity of the insect chemoreceptor is in the C_{11} to C_{12} aliphatic compounds of a given series. Trail pheromones (C_{16} to C_{18}), in which it is desirable to have a low threshold, a high specificity, but less volatility, fall slightly above this. Thus, the trail will persist long enough to be followed and be specific enough to be separated from other trails, yet it disappears at a rate sufficient to prevent residual false trails. On the other hand, the desirable qualities of an alarm pheromone would be rapid diffusion, a relatively wide broadcast range, and quick disappearance so that the source could be easily localized. Since these criteria are best fulfilled by a highly volatile compound, sensitivity and discrimination would best be sacrificed, which seems to be the case.

The ratio of pheromone molecules released to the response threshold concentrations (i.e., the alarm pheromone of *Po-*

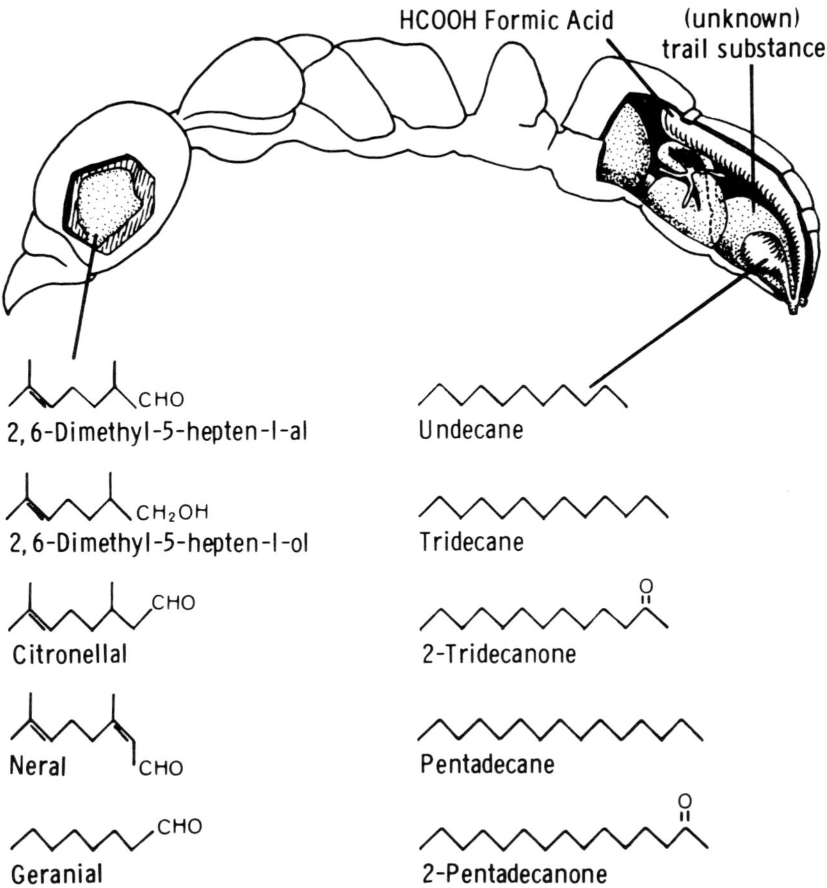

Figure 6. Location and nature of pheromones. (Modified from Wilson [3].)

gonomyrmex badius, 4-methyl-3-heptanone) lies between that of the sex attractant of moths (undecane, which could produce an active space measured in kilometers and persisting for years) and the fire ant trail substance at the other end of the spectrum which has a very limited active space but longer persistence than the alarm pheromone. There is no evidence of positive feedback of alarm pheromones; thus, this also aids in the localizing of signals.

Sex pheromone.—The sex pheromone has never been chemically identified but is presumed to exist since a similar chemical is known to exist in the bee. It is difficult to think of any other mechanism by which aerial mating could occur since the female follows after a time lag without visual contact with the male and yet finds him flying at about 200 m elevation. Attempts to demonstrate the existence of a sex pheromone have been unsuccessful thus far. Flights occurring in captive colonies do not result in fertilization, and this could possibly be related to the existence of baroreceptors for the altitude at which mating usually occurs. Attempts to simulate this elevation by evacuating a chamber did not result in mating (12).

Learning and Memory

The ant's capacity for learning is quite impressive considering its limited number of neural circuits. Workers of *Formica* spp. are able to learn a 6-point maze at a rate only two to three times slower than the laboratory rat (Fig. 7). It has also been shown that they can remember their way through these mazes for a period of up to 4 days (52, 53). They are also able simultaneously to memorize the position of four separate landmarks and remember them well enough to use them in orientation as long as 1 week later (54). It was first noted in bees that a worker (who had been searching in a tortuous pattern) upon encountering a food source would return by the shortest direct route, the beeline, to the nest. This same phenomenon has been demonstrated in the ant. In order to accomplish this, the ant must "calculate" the angle of deviation and the distance traveled and in essence "integrate" the area under the curves in order to arrive at a true straight line return. A human would require a stopwatch, compass, and calculus to accomplish this maneuver.

Lest one become overwhelmed with the apparent intelligence of

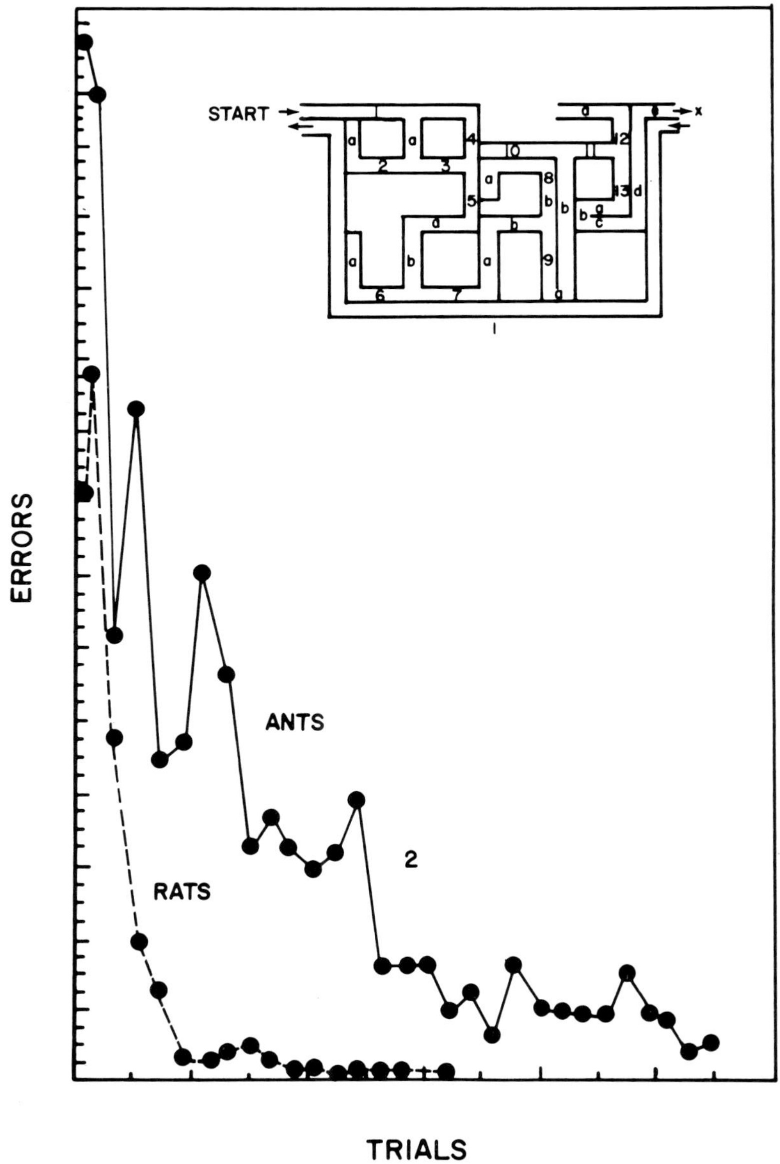

Figure 7. Maze learning by the ant. (Modified from Wilson [3].)

this creature, it seems appropriate to mention some of its limitations. Histological examination of the insect nervous system reveals a limited number of neurons with many dendritic arborations and connections. Due to the thinness of the myelin sheath and the lack of medullation, they conduct at about one-tenth the speed of vertebrate neurons. From these observations, Vowles (38) states: "The properties of the insect neuron and the small size of the insect nervous system render necessary functional organization far simpler than is often supposed. . . . What should arouse our wonder is the success with which simplicity has been crowned." Limitations include the fact that learning cannot have much of an abstract quality; it must be pertinent to the task at hand and to natural conditions. The ant has a very limited ability to transfer memory to new situations and almost no ability to generalize from experience. Thus, when a *Formica* worker is required to run a maze in reverse, even though it is proficient at running it in a forward direction, it treats it as an entirely new problem. The basic concept which emerges and helps to explain ant behavior is that the template of synaptic junctions is largely a printed circuit of programmed behavior with a limited ability to be modulated by a new experience. This hypothesis becomes attractive when one considers the large amount of stereotyped behavior exhibited by the ants. Second, it gives a better understanding of pheromones as releasers, or triggers, of such programmed behavior. Blocks of inherited behavior can be stimulated by chemical triggers with a certain allowance for learned behavior to modify these programs.

3

VENOM

The venom of the fire ant group is extremely unique. The venoms of most other poisonous arthropods and vertebrates are protein-based and are generally concentrated protein solutions (56–58). In fact, there is a great deal more similarity between bee venom and rattlesnake venom than between fire ant venom and bee venom (see Table 4).

The reason that this side road in the evolution of venoms is so unique is that some of the alkaloids contained in the fire ant venom are found nowhere else in the animal world and are a radical departure from the majority of venoms. Historically, the first major article to shed light on the subject was published in 1957 by Caro, Derbes, and Jung (59), who demonstrated the histological evolution of the skin lesion caused by intentional fire ant stings in volunteers. They also reported the first cases of systemic allergic reactions to the imported fire ant. In 1959, Adrouny, Derbes, and Jung (60, 61) isolated a crystallizable substance, which they designated Solamine. It was soluble in nonpolar solvents, gave a negative ninhydrin reaction, had marked hemolytic activity, and when injected into rabbit skin produced a reaction indistinguishable from the natural sting of the imported fire ant.

In 1958, Blum et al. (62) described a simple milking technique which involved holding the ant by the petiole, everting the stinger, and collecting the droplets of venom in a 1 μl capillary tube (under a dissecting microscope).[1] This obviated the previous

1. We have found this technique even more productive if the front portion of the ant is removed immediately prior to milking, thus preventing the legs from interfering with the milking procedure.

TABLE 4. COMPARISON OF IMPORTED FIRE ANT VENOM AND OTHER VENOMS

	Bee	Wasp	Elapids (Cobra)	Crotilidae (Rattlesnake)	Fire Ant
Basic composition	Protein	Protein	Protein	Protein	Non-protein
Major component	Mellitin (50%)				Alkaloid (95%)
Biogenic amines	Histamine	Histamine			None known
Enzymes	Phospholipase A PLB (?) Hyaluronidase	PLA PLB Hyaluronidase	PLA Hyaluronidase Proteases[a] DNAse RNAse ATPase (many other lytic enzymes)	PLA Hyaluronidase Proteases[b] DNAse RNAse ATPase Acetylcholine esterase Acid phosphatase (several more lytic enzymes)	None known
Toxins	Mellitin Mast cell degranulating substance	Wasp kinin			Alkaloid Hemolytic (58) Complement activation (71) Insecticidal (58) Bactericidal (63, 67)
Neurotoxins	Apamin		Cobratoxin (cobra) Bungarotoxins (Taiwan Krait)	Crotamine (rattlesnake)	Alkaloid Insect paralysis (63) Nerve depolarization (68)
Cardiotoxins			Cobra cardiotoxin		

SOURCE: Russell (56) and Minton (57).
a. Major Component.
b. Minor Component.

arduous procedure of individual gland dissection under magnification.[2] In the same study, Blum also reported the venom to be ninhydrin negative, indicating the absence of protein. He reaffirmed that the venom was insoluble in water but soluble in nonpolar solvents (62). He stated that the alkalinity of the mixture was due to metal ions and did some preliminary infrared and ultraviolet spectrum photometric examinations of this substance. He found the venom to be toxic to the fruit fly and several other insects and mites. Interestingly, he found that the fire ant was not highly susceptible to its own venom. The fire ant venom produced instantaneous paralysis in the tested insects, which he felt was suggestive of the effects of a nerve poison. Blum, MacConnell, Fales, and Brand (64–66) subsequently identified a component which they designated Solenopsin A. They studied it extensively with infrared spectrophotometry and mass spectrometry and defined its structure as a piperidine nucleus with a methylation of the 2 position and a 12 to 16 carbon aliphatic chain in the sixth position (Fig. 8). Subsequent studies (64, 67) have shown that this model holds for all of the species of the *Solenopsis* group. All of the differences discovered between the species were in the side chain, either in the number of carbons or in the number or arrangement of double bonds and stereoisomers. Moreover, they found that the particular type and ratio of alkaloids was characteristic of the given species (Fig. 9) and that these patterns could be used to identify the species. This constancy further substantiated Buren's (7) taxonomic reclassification.

The taxonomy of this group had been difficult and speculation on the order of evolution even more confusing. By analyzing the alkaloid components of the venoms, Brand and Blum (67) were able to present a logical argument for establishing the evolution of the *Solenopsis* group; this argument, however, is not universally accepted (7).

Venom taken from the workers of *S. xyloni* and *S. geminata* contained varying ratios of *cis*-11 and *trans*-11, 2-methyl-6-n-undecylpiperidine (where it was the major compound with

2. A further possible improvement on this technique has been the use of electroshock to get the ant to extrude venom into a small depression in a plate (63). This is the first time that this technique has been described, although a similar technique of electrical grid stimulation has been used to obtain bee venom for quite some time.

only trace amounts of the C_{13} compounds). The *cis* and *trans* C_{11} compounds were also found in *S. richteri* and *S. invicta* but were minor components. In addition, the predominant isomer was the *trans* isomer. In *S. richteri*, the C_{13} compounds predominated and the *trans* form of all components predominated.

The venom of *S. invicta* proved to be the most complex. It contained all of the previous components with a marked predominance of the *trans* isomers and, in addition, was the only venom containing *cis* and *trans* C_{15} compounds. Thus, the venoms of *S. xyloni* and *S. geminata* seem very similar with a predominance of *cis* isomers. The *S. richteri* and *S. invicta* venoms are progressively more complex with a marked predominance of the *trans* isomer (see Fig. 9).

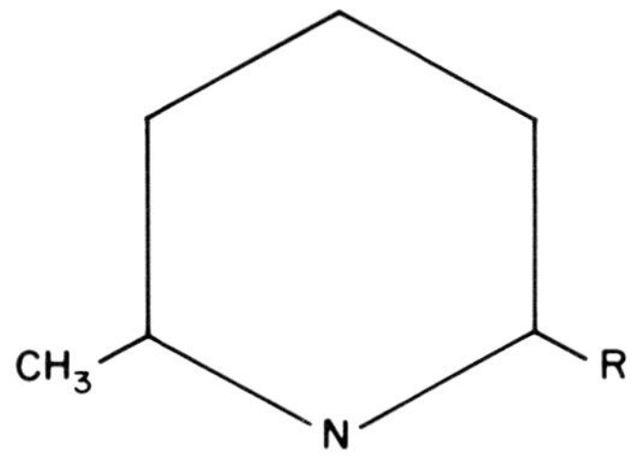

R = ① $CH_2 \cdot (CH_2)_9 \cdot CH_3$
TRANS-2-METHYL-6-N-UNDECYLPIPERIDINE

R = ② $(CH_2)_3\,\overset{H}{C}=\overset{H}{C}-(CH_2)_7CH_3$
TRANS-2-METHYL-6-(CIS-4-TRIDECYL)PIPERIDINE

R = ③ $CH_2(CH_2)_{13}\,CH_3$
TRANS-2-METHYL-6-N-PENTADECYLPIPERIDINE

Figure 8. Structure of alkaloid. (Courtesy of Blum: *Tetrahedron* 26:1129–39, 1971.)

Analysis showed that the venoms from the winged queens of all species were essentially the same. They contained only C_{11} compounds in slightly different ratios but with a continuous predominance of the *cis* isomer (67). Brand and Blum argued that the predominant *cis* C_{11} form found in all the queens and in the workers of *S. xyloni* and *S. geminata* was the primitive state and that *S. richteri* and *S. invicta* represented a more complex and a more highly evolved state.

There are several other lines of reasoning which would support this conclusion. *S. invicta* has been shown experimentally and clinically to have the most toxic venom. It seems reasonable to believe that a more effective venom would represent a more highly evolved state with greater survival value. Brand and Blum presented several additional arguments which also support this conclusion:

1. *S. geminata* is the only member of the fire ant group that has a true soldier caste. Since soldiers occur commonly throughout the subfamily Myrmicinae from which *Solenopsis* is derived, this could be considered an ancestral trait (controversial).

2. Thermodynamically, the easiest combination to synthesize is

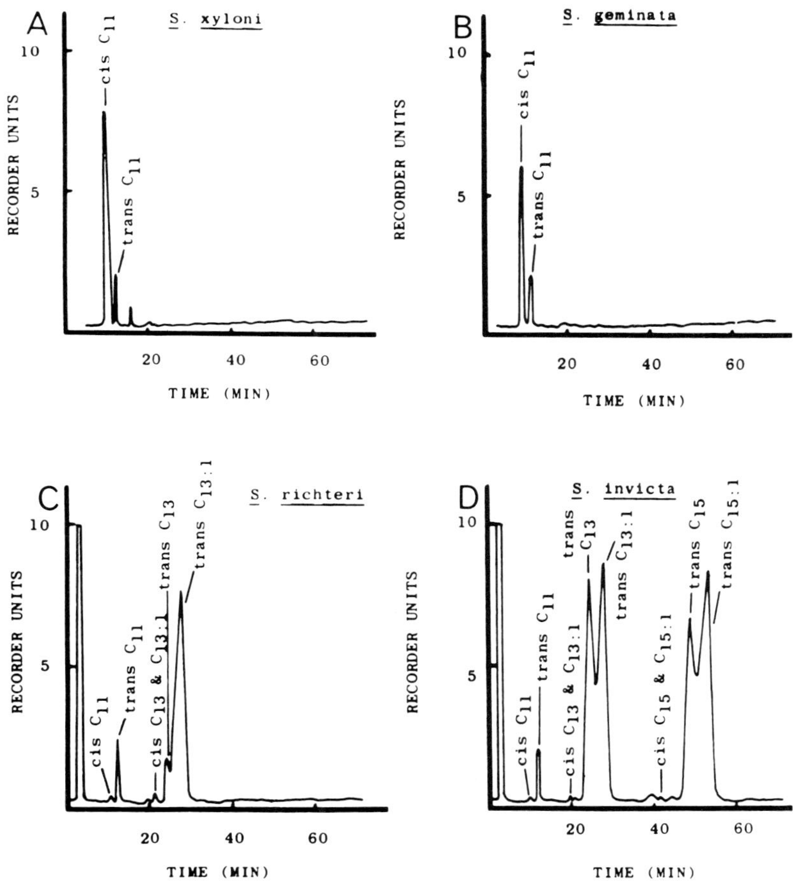

Figure 9. Gas chromatograms of the venom alkaloids from worker ants of four species of fire ant.

that of *S. xyloni* and *S. geminata* with a marked predominance of the *cis* isomer. It is thermodynamically more difficult and requires the addition of two more enzymes to create the compounds found in the *S. richteri* and *S. invicta* lines. This would be in keeping with progressive evolution.

3. The similarity of the venoms of the queens of all species to that of *geminata* and *xyloni* is considered to be a representation of the primal state. They reasoned from this that there would be a positive pressure for evolution of a more effective venom on the part of the soldiers, while the queen was protected by the entire colony. It would therefore follow that there was no selective pressure on her to develop a more effective venom (also controversial).

Brand and Blum also proposed an explanation for the increased toxicity of the *S. invicta* venom as compared to that of *S. xyloni* and *S. geminata*. The characteristic finding in the *richteri* and *invicta* of a more highly unsaturated side chain and a switch to the *trans* configuration both favor increased polarity of the molecule. Such polarity would favor exposure of an electron pair of the nitrogen atom. The unsaturated *trans* isomer with its slightly polar character would make it better able to dissolve in lipophilic substances such as insect cuticle and inter- and intracellular membranes. After penetrating, these exposed nitrogen electrons would represent a likely point of attack (67).

An additional interesting sideline of this research into the alkaloid components of the fire ant venom is the observation that within an *S. geminata* colony there is the variable ratio of *cis* to *trans* isomer of a C_{11} compound. However, if the *cis* to *trans* ratio is plotted against the head length in millimeters, it produces a linear relationship the slope of which is characteristic of a given colony. In one of the colonies studied the data best fit into two separate lines with significantly different slopes. It was reasoned from this that the colony contained two functional queens (18).

Currently described physiologic properties of the venom alkaloid include hemolytic (60) and insecticidal activities (62). In addition, several studies have shown direct tissue toxicity caused by this alkaloid which faithfully reproduces the changes of the natural sting (61, 68).[3] Its tissue reaction resembles in some ways

3. This activity, however, has been shown to be limited to 4 of 7 alkaloids tested in rabbit skin: *cis* C_{11}, *trans* C_{13}, *cis* C_{15}, and *cis* $C_{15:1}$ (68).

that of the brown recluse spider *Loxosceles reclusus*. In addition, bactericidal activity has been documented which helps explain the sterility of the pustules formed (62, 69). The effect of the alkaloid on neurotransmission in standard neurophysiologic preparations has been studied by Buffkin and Russell (68, 70) with negative results There is other work, however, indicating some interference with neurotransmission. In a preparation of end plate membrane of frog skeletal muscle, suppression of AcCh sensitivity similar to that caused by a tubocurarine has been shown. At higher concentrations, the alkaloid depolarizes the membrane (71).

An additional rather serendipitous finding has been that the fire ant venom alkaloids appear to cause activation of the alternate complement pathway (72). This is currently being investigated. The experiment was originally predicated on the assumption that fire ant venom was something like cobra venom, which is known to de-complement serum. Because of the simple nature of the chemical and the proposed activity of the nitrogen electron pair, this could be a powerful tool in the elucidation of the alternate complement pathway and may also help to explain its local tissue toxicity.

Although Blum (46) has noted that on centrifugation of the whole venom there was a small aqueous component comprising about 5 percent of the total volume, he was not able to accumulate much data about this fraction. Buffkin and Russell (68, 70), in addition to doing some studies on neurological systems, also did some preliminary investigations of this aqueous phase. They prepared a butanol extract of whole venom and found 7 amino acid residues in this fraction. On paper strip electrophoresis, samples of macerated venom glands extracted with saline revealed 2 peptide bands felt to be in the range of 6,000–12,000 molecular weight, which migrated towards the cathode.

The immunology of the fire ant venom and the nature of the allergen involved has been little studied. Russell attempted to sensitize rabbits to the fire ant venom, but was unsuccessful. In view of the known lack of persistence of serum reagent antibody in the rabbit, this is not surprising (73). Therapy of fire ant hypersensitivity with whole body extract injections was empirically based on an extrapolation (made in blissful ignorance) of the data from the therapy of the other stinging hymenoptera. However, since the only available model for this therapy is this data, let us explore it further. Foubert and Stier (74) reported that the honeybee, polistes wasp, hornet, and yellow jacket contained 4–6 antigenic components as demonstrated by gel diffusion. They further reported that 2 of the antigens were common between the bee and the yellow jacket. They proposed that these shared antigens could serve as the basis for the clinically observed cross-sensitivity among the various species. There was disagreement among various authors about the number of fractions present and the degree of cross-reactivity probably related to different methods used for identification (74–79). In general, those using immunoelectrophoresis demonstrated more fractions (9–13) than those using gel immunodiffusion (76). There is general agreement among the authors, however, that the venom sac contained fewer components than the whole body and that the pure venom contains even fewer components. In a series of papers, Arbesman et al. (75, 77, 78) presented results of chromotography of whole body and venom sac extracts from the bee, hornet, and yellow jacket. They demonstrated that skin test reactivity resided in only certain of the column fractions and that there were two types of fractions producing skin test reactivity, namely, species-specific antigens and cross-reacting antigens. Their conclusions were as follows: specific antigens for each type of insect were isolated from whole insect and venom sac extracts; the species-specific antigens always gave the highest titers by skin test in sensitive patients; the species-specific antigen with the highest allergenic activity was distributed in the venom sac and the body of the insect; each type of insect contains one or more different antigens which control the antigenic relationship with the other two species of insects and which induce allergenic reactions in human beings; and the cross-reacting antigens with allergenic activity were apparently localized in the insect body and not found in the venom sac extracts.

The final point is the one on which there has been the most debate, i.e., the presence and number of cross-reacting antigens in venom (79). A study with purified venom, using immunodiffusion techniques demonstrated cross-reacting action antigens in the venoms of the polistes wasp, yellow jacket, yellow hornet, and honeybee and showed species-specific antigens in each of these venoms (80). Lichtenstein, Valentine, and Sobotka (81) have treated patients who are sensitive only to species-specific venom components.

There was no histamine release from basophiles (sensitized with patient serum) when challenged with whole body extracts of honeybee or mixed stinging insects. The same patient's serum caused marked basophile histamine release when challenged with honeybee venom. These patients were not protected clinically by injection therapy with whole body extract, but by honeybee venom immunotherapy (81). This newer data would give impetus to the use of purified venom initially introduced by Loveless (82) a number of years ago. The clinical data that have been collected by the Insect Allergy Committee of the American Academy of Allergy weigh heavily in the other direction. The accumulated data would indicate a greater than 95 percent protection rate from allergic reactions to stinging hymenoptera with the use of whole body extract immunotherapy (79, 83). This would support the concept that the patient sensitive to a single species-specific venom component represents a special case.

In the case of the imported fire ant, there is a clinical suggestion of cross-reactivity (see chapter 4). The vast difference between the highly concentrated proteinaceous bee and wasp venom and the basically alkaloid venom of the fire ant with only a trace of protein does not encourage making analogies between the two. If one does pursue this analogy, however, the explanation for the apparent clinical cross-sensitivity would rest in a cross-reacting body protein between fire ants and the other hymenoptera. This shared antigenic component would have to be present in the fire ant venom.

In order to examine the first part of this hypothesis, we immunized a series of rabbits to whole body extracts of various hymenoptera, including *S. invicta* and *S. richteri*. The results of gel immunodiffusion using these hyperimmune serums are shown in Figures 10 and 11. There was some degree of cross-reactivity between the fire ant species and honeybee, hornet, and yellow jacket but not the polistes wasp. Making use of the fact that rabbit gamma-2 IgG (nonreaginic) antibody binds to guinea pig mass cells, 6-hour PCA's (Passive Cutaneous Anaphylaxis) were carried out, using these hyperimmune rabbit serums. These results tended to confirm those of the gel diffusion as is shown in Figures 12 and 13.

Spence (84), using a similar experimental system, demonstrated (by gel diffusion and 6-hour PCA's) cross-reactions between fire ant whole body extract, venom, and purified Solamine (alkaloid). This showed that the alkaloid was present in propylene glycol venom and whole body extracts in sufficient amounts to be demonstrated by immunologic means.[4] The experiment did not shed any light on the allergenicity of the alkaloid.

These data could serve as an explanation of the apparent clinical cross-sensitivity between the imported fire ant and other hymenoptera, if the same antigen could be shown to be present in the fire ant venom. Experiments to answer this question are currently underway in our laboratory. If this is indeed the allergen of the fire ant venom, it must be extremely potent, since the sting of a single fire ant can produce anaphylaxis, the sting volume of the fire ant (estimated by Blum [18] to be 0.007–0.11 μl in *S. geminata*)[5] is miniscule compared to that of the bee or the yellow jacket, and the protein content of fire ant venom is less than 1 percent as compared with the protein content of honeybee venom

ANTIGEN \ ANTIBODY	S. Invicta	S. Ricterii	Black Ant	Invicta (sting)	Yellow Jacket	Hornet	Wasp	Honey Bee	Honey Bee Venom	Phospholipase A
S. Invicta	+	+	-	-	+	+	+	+	-	
S. Richterii	+	+	-	-	+	+	-	+	-	
Black Ant	-	-	-		-	-	-	-		
Yellow Jacket	-	-	-	-	+	+	-	+	-	
Hornet	-	-	-		-	+	-	-	-	
Wasp	-	-	-	-	+	+	+	+	-	
Honey Bee	+	+			+	-	+	-	-	
Honey Bee Venom	-	-	-		-	-	-	-	+	

Figure 10. Results of gel diffusion tests.

4. There is no evidence, nor is it theoretically probable, that there is any significant amount of alkaloid in commercial saline extracts of whole fire ants.

5. In our experience, a microliter tube can be filled by milking 10–20 *S. invicta* major workers.

which is greater than 40 percent. The only other potential sources of the allergen, if it is not present in the aqueous phase, would primarily be the predominant alkaloid phase, in which case it would have to be a hapten, as has been suggested (68). The final possibility is speculative, but the fire ant, as well as the other

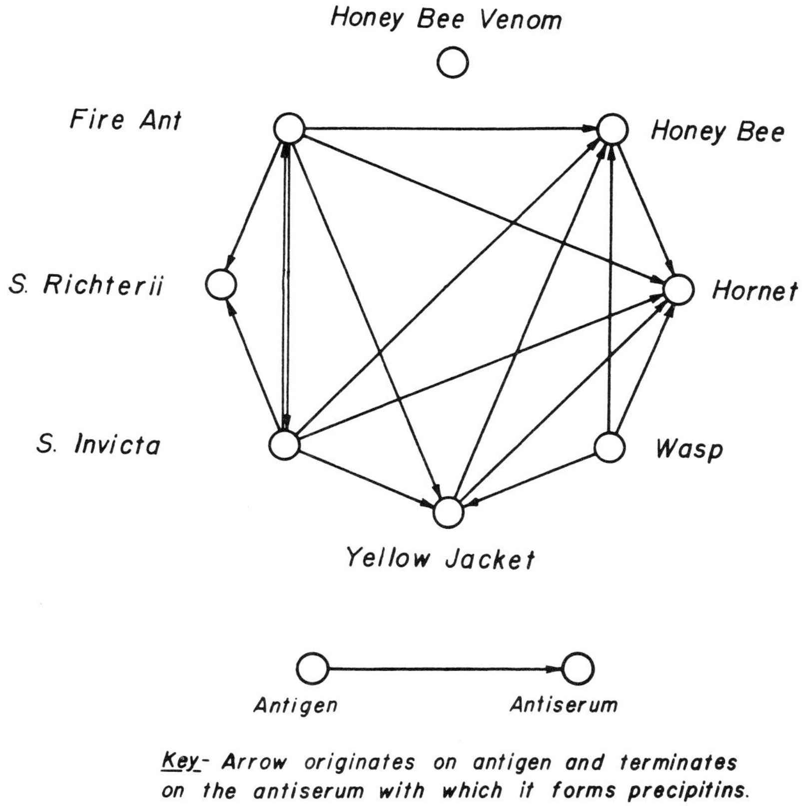

Figure 11. Cross-reactions of hymenoptera whole body extracts, using gel immunodiffusion.

stinging hymenoptera, has a peculiar mandibular groove and modified salivary apparatus which could serve as a venom gland for introduction of an allergen (85).

We are attempting to answer this question by preparing a number of fractions to be used in skin testing of new imported-fire-ant-sensitive patients. This includes a saline body extract

ANTIGEN \ ANTIBODY	S. Invicta	S. Ricterii	Black Ant	Invicta (sting)	Yellow Jacket	Hornet	Wasp	Honey Bee	Honey Bee Venom	Phospholipase A
S. Invicta	+	+	+	-	+	-	+	-		
S. Richterii	+	+	+		-	-	-	-	-	-
Black Ant	-	-	+		-	-	+	-	-	-
Yellow Jacket	-	-			+	+	+	+		
Hornet	-	-	+	-	+	+	+	+		
Wasp	-	-			+	+	+	+		
Honey Bee	-	-	-		+	-	-	-	+	-
Honey Bee Venom										

Figure 12. Results of PCA testing.

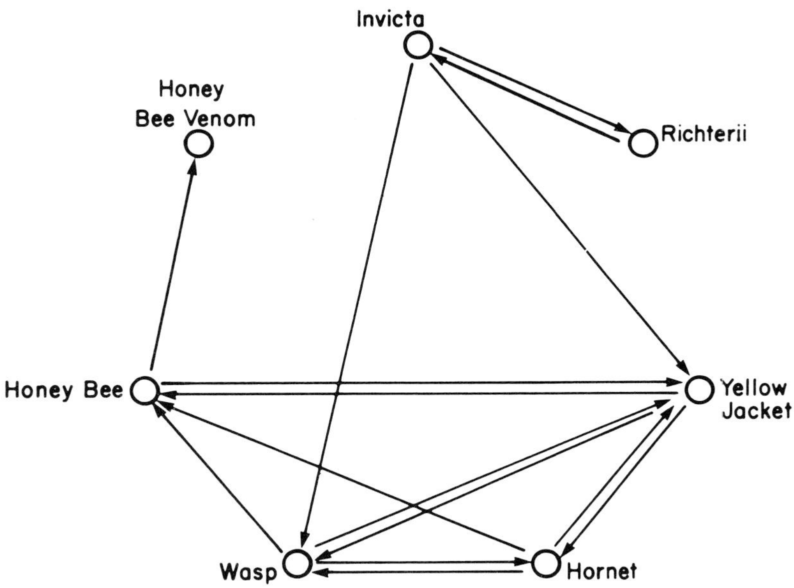

Figure 13. Cross-reactions of hymenoptera whole body extracts, using passive cutaneous anaphylaxis with hyperimmune rabbit sera in pigs.

prepared from fire ant front halves by standard methods. In addition, the venom of over 3,000 *S. invicta* workers was obtained by the milking technique of Blum et al. (62). This venom was then centrifuged, separating the alkaloid and aqueous phases. The capillary tubes were broken off at the line of demarcation between the two phases and the two samples were extracted separately. Synthetic alkaloid was generously supplied by Dr. Blum. It is hoped that by skin testing with these components, the location of the allergenic component can be identified.

If the antigen responsible for the allergic reactions to the fire ant stings can be identified, it will be possible to take a more informed approach toward therapy. James et al. (86) have found that whole venom contains marked skin reactivity. Our preliminary results indicate that this skin test reactivity resides in the aqueous phase rather than in the alkaloid phase.

In March 1977, Dr. Harold Baer of the FDA presented an abstract, "Fire Ant Allergy: Isolation of Three Allergenic Proteins from Whole Venom." Using nonpolar extraction, then column fractionation of the aqueous phase, his lab identified 3 protein fractions from the aqueous phase of *S. invicta* venom. These proteins (minimum molecular weights 10,000, 5,000, 2,000) were shown to be allergenic by skin test and RAST determinations with IFA-allergic patients and their serums. Amino acid analysis of the fractions (95, 50, and 20 amino acids, respectively) confirmed that they were distinct and separate proteins. There was some suggestion that one of the fractions may have phospholipase activity. All patients tested reacted to at least one of the fractions.

This study clearly places the allergen in the aqueous phase and allows possible explanation of the cross reactivity, but raises the question of the extreme potency of this antigen since it is presented in such small amounts.

4

CLINICAL DATA

Although the terms "bite" and "sting" have been used interchangeably, the attack mechanism of this ant should be mentioned. The imported fire ant does indeed bite with its jaws, but this is thought to be primarily for the purpose of securing itself to the victim. It then proceeds to pivot about its head, stinging at multiple sites in a circular distribution with its abdominal stinger which is a modified ovapositor with associated venom gland.

The sting of the imported fire ant produces a sterile pustule within 24 hours (Fig. 14). This is a very significant diagnostic finding since for all practical purposes this is the only insect in the United States whose sting produces a pustule of this type. The absence of a pustule does not, however, exclude the possibility of a sting of the imported fire ant (7). Pustules are occasionally caused by the sting of *S. xyloni* (59, 87).

If one finds a true, intact pustule present 18–24 hours after the bite, there is really no differential diagnosis. The bite of the blister beetle is a true bullous lesion, not a pustule. Secondarily infected stings or bites are generally on a larger, more inflamed base and appear later than 24 hours. The venom of the brown recluse spider, *Loxosceles reclusus*, although also causing direct tissue necrosis, does not cause a lesion resembling that caused by the imported fire ant.

HISTOPATHOLOGY

Caro, Derbes, and Jung (59) studied the development of cutaneous lesions with the aid of volunteers who permitted themselves to be stung by the imported fire ant. Biopsy specimens were removed at 6 minutes, 30 minutes, 24 hours, and 72 hours after the stings occurred. In a section removed from the sting site at 6 minutes, the epidermis showed no pathological changes. There was edema in the upper corium and narrow mantles of lymphocytes and histiocytes about the superficial capillaries.

At 30 minutes, the section showed considerable edema throughout the epidermis, mostly of the intracellular type. The basal layer was intact, but markedly edematous. The superficial blood vessels were dilated and surrounded by a slight infiltrate of

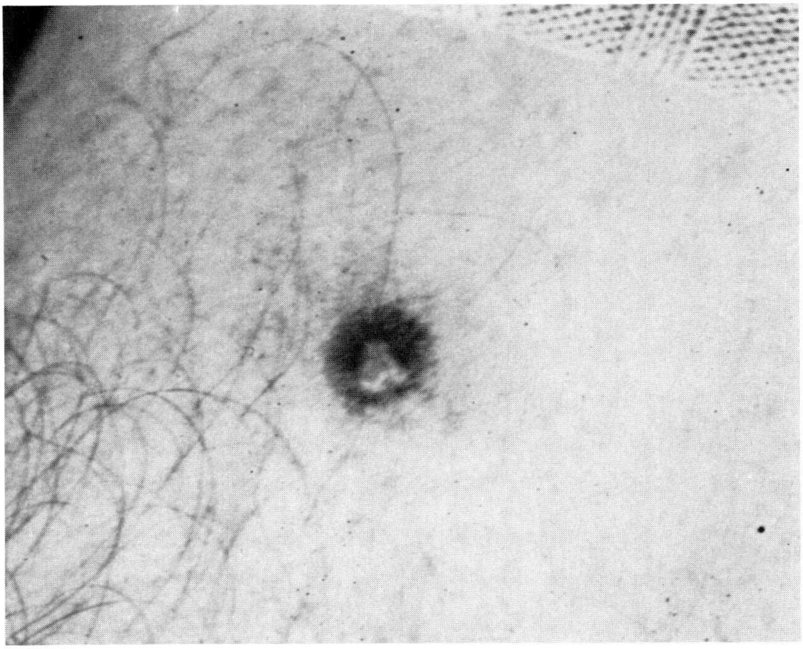

Figure 14. Fire ant pustule. (Courtesy of Greer Laboratories.)

lymphocytes, histiocytes, and plasma cells. In the upper corium, there were several irregularly shaped but well-outlined masses of early necrosis in which the connective tissue fibers were amorphous and stained poorly.

At 24 hours, the lesion was a superficial pustule; the roof was thin and composed of a thin, horny layer and a layer of a few epidermal cells. The sides of the pustule were rounded and distinctly demarcated from the adjoining epidermis. The contents included many necrotic polymorphonuclear lymphocytes. The floor consisted of densely packed necrotic connective tissue, beneath which lay a diffuse infiltrate of polymorphonuclear leukocytes, lymphocytes, and cells with small pyknotic nuclei that permeated the poorly stained connective tissue and surrounded the blood vessels.

At 72 hours, the pustule was still intact, but the roof was very thin. At this time, the pustule contained many eosinophilic leukocytes and plasma cells, in addition to the cells noted above. The floor of the pustule consisted of an edematous epidermis everywhere except at the center. In this central area, the epidermal floor was completely absent, and the cellular infiltrate broke through to extend profusely into the underlying necrotic connective tissue. Mantles of cellular infiltrate also extended laterally and more deeply about the dilated blood vessels and about the nearby sweat glands. Numerous cultures of the pustules produced, with one exception, negative results. On one occasion, nonhemolytic staphylococci were grown, but organisms were not seen in tissue removed for biopsy.

These histopathologic changes were not of the type generally seen after other insect stings and bites. Caro, Derbes, and Jung (59) stated that the inflammatory reaction was much more severe, the consistent formation of a pustule was a differentiating feature, and the necrosis often led to scar production.

Materials and Results

We have recently completed an analysis of the combined experience of 11 practicing allergists in the state of Florida (88).[1] The results follow.

All patients had a history of a reaction of the immediate type involving a part of the body distant from the site of the sting. Patients with exaggerated local reactions only, even those with swelling across neighboring joints, were excluded. Patients with systemic reactions to unspecified ants in which documentation of fire ant involvement could not be accomplished were also excluded.

Either pustule formation at the sting site or a positive skin test

1. Drs. Robert B. Rhoades, Walter L. Schafer, William H. Schmid, Paul F. Wubbena, Richard M. Dozier, Andrew W. Townes, M. Newman, G. Neder, R. Lockey, T. Brill, and Heinz J. Wittig.

for the imported fire ant, or both, served as presumptive evidence of specificity for the imported fire ant. Six of the cases were further confirmed by identification of the offending ants as *S. invicta* by Buren (7).

Clinical data are summarized in Tables 5–7, and treatment results are shown in Table 8.

Patients whose initial visit to the participating allergists was between October 1973 and November 1974 were separated in order to analyze the frequency of the problem. Jacksonville, Florida, was chosen as the prime area for analysis because: it is served almost entirely by two allergists, Drs. Newman and

TABLE 5. HISTORIES OF FIRE ANT HYPERSENSITIVITY

	Number	Percent
Number of patients	104	100
Male	52/104	50
Female	52/104	50
Age (1–72 years)	23 yrs [a]	
Children (0–18 years)	44/104	42
Time of onset of symptoms (1–60 min)	13 min [a]	
Number of bites (1–100)	10[a]	
History of allergy	28/83	34
History of other insect sensitivity	8/104	7
History of systemic reaction to previous ant bites	19/104	18
Pustules present at 24 hrs	62/72	86
Pustules not present at 24 hrs	10/72	14

a. Average.

Wubbena, both of whom participated in the study; it is a large population center surrounded by an area which is basically rural with no competing center offering this service within a 50-mile radius; and based on observations of USDA entomologists, the fire ant infestation can be considered moderate and representative of many other areas in the state (12). A limited analysis was also done to estimate the incidence rate over the last few years in certain selected allergy practices (which are fairly stable) to determine whether there was any trend in the incidence of the fire ant hypersensitivity. The patient charts of one busy practice were analyzed and a comparison was made of the incidence of other ant-stinging hymenoptera sensitivity and fire ant sensitivity.

As seen in Table 5, 8 patients had associated hypersensitivity reactions to other insects. These included 1 mild to moderate generalized reaction to deerfly, 1 severe systemic reaction to the saddleback caterpillar, 1 severe reaction to spider bite, and 5 patients with systemic reaction to bee, hornet, or wasp stings.

TABLE 6. Signs and Symptoms of Fire Ant Hypersensitivity

	Number	Percent
Skin		
Generalized urticaria	80	77
Generalized angioedema	70	67
Respiratory		
Tightness in chest	17	16
Difficulty breathing	30	29
Wheezing	14	14
Cough	10	10
"Could not talk"	5	5
Chest pain	11	11
Hoarseness	6	6
Laryngeal edema	1	1
GI		
Nausea	11	11
Vomiting	5	5
Abdominal pain	6	6
Dysphagia	7	7
Swollen throat or tongue	3	3
Itching throat	1	1
Choking	3	3
Cardiovascular		
Fall in blood pressure	11	10
Collapse	13	12
Dizziness	20	19
Sweating	10	10
Cyanosis	3	3
Vasoconstriction or vasodilation	6	6
Tachycardia and palpitations	2	2
Neurologic		
Unconsciousness	11	11
Convulsions	3	3
Blurred vision	2	2
Confusion	1	1
Drowsiness	2	2
General		
Malaise	1	1
Fever	2	2
Head throbbing	1	1
Weakness	3	3
Leg pains	1	1
Generalized pruritus	13	12
Numbness	1	1

The patients with stinging-hymenoptera sensitivity were also treated with aqueous extract of mixed stinging insects.

The highest estimated number of stings was 100, so that the possibility of systemic reactions on the basis of venom toxicity could be eliminated. Other authors have noted the occurrence of hundreds of stings in nonsensitive individuals without systemic symptoms (7, 89, 90). The times of onset of symptoms after the sting ranged from 1 to 60 minutes, thus excluding cases of delayed onset reactions. The presence or absence of pustules was documented in 69 percent of the patients. Of these, 86 percent

TABLE 7. Skin Test Results of Fire Ant Hypersensitivity in 86 Patients

To Fire Ant	Scratch	ID
1:10,000,000		5
1:1,000,000	1	6
1:100,000	1	12
1:10,000	3	15[a]
1:1,000	2	15[b]
1:100	6	1
1:20	15	
Negative skin test: 4 patients		
Other stinging hymenoptera		
Wasp		
Yellow jacket		
Bee		
Hornet		
Red ant		
Positive: 17/39		

a. Or 100 PNU.
b. Or 1,000 PNU.

had pustules. All other patients had positive skin test reactions to aqueous extracts of the imported fire ant.

There were four instances of the systemic reactions from skin testing. One man reported moderate substernal pain following scratch testing, and one child experienced generalized urticaria within 15 minutes after a positive scratch test. A third man developed itching of the armpit within 10 minutes of intradermal skin test on that arm, and a fourth man developed hives and pruritus shortly after skin testing.

As seen in Table 8, 92 of 104 patients received hyposensitizing injection therapy. Of 19 patients re-stung after beginning therapy, only 2 had constitutional reactions. All other patients had only local reactions. The hyposensitization schedules varied, but all of them began with weekly injections at the approximate level of sensitivity shown on the skin testing. Most of the patients listed in Table 8 were re-stung while on maintenance therapy, generally in the range of weekly injections of .5 cc of a 1:10 to a 1:50 weight:volume dilution of fire ant extract. Clearly, a number of individuals appeared to be protected by much lower concentra-

TABLE 8. Results of Hyposensitization Therapy in 19 Patients

Patient	Age	Sex	Duration of Treatment at Time of Re-sting[a]	Type of Reaction
W. S.	11	M	8 months	Local
P. R.	26	M	7 months	Local
D. D.	7	F	Off treatment one year	Local
A. B.	9	M	6 months	General (Case 2)
N. D.	42	F	3 months	Local
J. B.	33	M	6–18 months (stung on several occasions)	(see Chapter 4)
K. M.	27	F	1 year (re-stung 4 times)	Local (Case 1)
J. B.	2	M	2 years (multiple re-stings)	Local
J. F.	14	M	4 months (re-stung 3 times)	Local
W. B.	50	M	6 months (multiple re-stings)	Local (Case 4)
C. H.	3	M	4 months (1 episode; 4 bites)	Local
B. T.	30	F	1 month (1 bite on 2 occasions)	Local
S. P.	26	F	4 months (1 bite)	Local
J. B.	2.5	M	3–4 years (re-stung several times)	Local
D. P.	3	M	4 months (2 bites)	Local
M. R.	38	M	1–2 months (re-stung 2 times)	Local
M. L.	3	M	2 months	Local
I. M.	46	F	8 months	Local

Note: Number of patients treated, 92/104; number of patients re-stung after therapy, 19/92; number of systemic reactions while on therapy, 2/19.

a. All patients were treated with aqueous extracts obtained from Greer Laboratories, Inc., Lenoir, North Carolina.

tions. However, in view of the variability of response (discussed later), it is somewhat tenuous to speculate about amounts required for protection. About half of the patients had been re-stung on more than one occasion, resulting in only local reaction.

Incidence Data (Table 9)

An analysis of the patient charts from an allergist in Jacksonville revealed 772 new patient work-ups during the period from November 1, 1973, through October 31, 1974. Of these, there were 15 cases of systemic allergic reactions to the stinging hymenoptera (bees, wasps, hornets, yellow jackets, etc.), as compared to 18 cases of systemic allergic reactions to fire ant stings. The samplings tend to support the impression of several other allergists throughout the central and northern parts of the state that the incidence of imported fire ant hypersensitivity approaches or exceeds the incidence of allergic reactions of the other hymenoptera combined.

The data from 6 allergists throughout the state were collected for the entire period prior to October 1973 via a retrospective

TABLE 9. INCIDENCE OF SYSTEMIC ALLERGIC REACTIONS TO THE IMPORTED FIRE ANT (NEW CASES)

Incidence in allergy practice[a] of imported fire ant and other hymenoptera sensitivity			
Jacksonville, Florida (11/1/73–10/31/74)			
Total new patients			772
Imported-fire-ant-sensitive patients			18
Other hymenoptera-sensitive patients			15
Tampa, Florida			
Total new patients			500
Imported-fire-ant-sensitive patients			15
Other hymenoptera-sensitive patients			10
Incidence of new imported-fire-ant-sensitivity cases over time in stable practice			
	Prior to 1972	10/72–10/73	11/73–10/74
St. Petersburg, Florida	5	7	8
Tallahassee, Florida	7	6	3
Minimal incidence per population area served			
Jacksonville		21 cases/year = 3.8/100,000/year	

a. All practices are of full-time allergists.

record search. A number of the members of this group had been in the same practice for more than 5 years and one of them for over 15 years; this search produced 49 cases. Cases recorded between November 1, 1973, and October 31, 1974, included two new major contributors (Drs. Newman and Lockey) whose records were not analyzed prior to November 1973. Excluding their cases, there are 25 cases from the original contributors in one year, as compared to twice that number in their combined practice experience prior to November 1, 1973. This is an impressive rise, even if we concede that some of it may be due to increased sensitivity to the diagnosis.

An analysis was performed in an attempt to get incidence figures. These figures represent minimal incidence of well-documented cases, because not all of the affected patients are seen by allergists. Therefore, the risk population is underestimated. There were 21 new cases in metropolitan Jacksonville during the year ending October 31, 1974. The population of the area was approximately 560,000 midway through the year used for calculation, giving an incidence of 3.8 new cases of imported fire ant sensitivity per 100,000 population per year.

Case Reports

Case 1.—K. M., a 27-year-old woman without previous allergic history, was bitten on August 18, 1972, by two ants on her right great toe. This produced local burning and itching, progressing in a matter of a few minutes to urticaria, dyspnea, chest pain, and general pruritus. When this increased over the next half hour to severe dyspnea with dizziness, she was admitted to the emergency room and diagnosed as being in anaphylactic shock with diminished blood pressure and unconsciousness. This condition responded to intravenous treatment with adrenalin and steroids and supportive measures. Two weeks prior to this episode she had received five stings which produced nausea and vertigo and a local reaction only. She had a 3+ intradermal skin test with 1 to 10 million dilution of Greer stock fire ant extract and a 2+ reaction to 1 to 1 million dilution of mixed stinging insects. She had no previous history of stinging insect sensitivity. Treatment was begun in August 1972 with aqueous fire ant extract. She has subsequently been re-stung on four occasions between August 2, 1973, and September 3, 1973 (twice with pustule formation), with no systemic symptoms at all.

This case is a good example of the severe life-threatening nature of the problem, the exquisite sensitivity demonstrated on the skin testing, and the apparent excellent results of hyposensitization therapy.

Case 2.—A. B. is a 9-year-old boy with a history of perennial allergic rhinitis and prior anaphylactic reaction to penicillin. At age 7 he developed a systemic allergic reaction to the sting of the imported fire ant. He had a 3+ reaction to intradermal skin testing with 1 to 1 million dilution of fire ant extract, but was negative to black ant extract. In addition to his immediate skin test reaction he also had a delayed reaction at the skin test site several hours later. He was started on injections of imported fire ant extract at a 1 to 3 million dilution in December 1972. Shortly after beginning injections he received a spider bite which resulted in immediate onset of dyspnea, cyanosis, and facial edema, requiring oxygen, adrenalin, and Decadron before resolving. In April 1973, while receiving weekly injections of .05 cc of 1 to 3 thousand dilution, he sustained several fire ant stings which resulted in immediate generalized angioedema which was treated with adrenalin and subsided. His dose of vaccine subsequently had to be reduced because of marked delayed local reactions to the injections. In September 1973, while receiving dosages of 0.5 cc of 1 to 30 thousand dilution, he sustained ant stings which produced pustules and a delayed reaction at the site, but no systemic effects. Again in November 1973, while receiving .3 cc of 1 to 30 thousand extract, he was stung and had local reactions only. To date he has been on vaccine for 2 years and has not been re-stung since November 1973.

Case 3.—F. B. is a 2-year-old boy without a previous history of allergy who, in July 1973, had 5 to 6 ant stings with pustule formation and no systemic symptoms. On August 31, 1973, he received approximately 30 stings on his legs and feet, causing pustule formation and the onset of generalized urticaria, coughing, and choking within 10 minutes. On September 9, 1973, he had one ant sting which resulted in pustule formation without associated systemic symptoms. He was being worked-up at the time and had not yet received hyposensitization therapy.

Case 4.—W. B. is an experienced ant taxonomist who had received many stings over a period of years from the domestic fire ant and other domestic ant species. In June 1968, he had his first exposure to *S. richteri*. Over a 2-hour period he received 20–30 stings, which produced multiple pustules. He then noted the onset of progressive generalized urticaria and angioedema along with the sensation of general malaise and tightness in his chest. He was taken to a local emergency room where his symptoms cleared after an injection of adrenalin. He then received 6 months of hyposensitization therapy during the remainder of 1968. Subsequent to that time he has had very rare episodes of 1 to 2 stings of the *S. richteri* species and many stings on multiple occasions from *S. invicta* without any systemic reaction. The question of the efficacy of that 6 months of therapy is a confusing one. The other question brought forth by his history is that of species specificity and cross-sensitivity. Since he reacted to his initial exposure to *S. richteri*, this would surely have been a cross-sensitivity from some other insect species to which he had previously been exposed. On the other hand, one might attribute his lack of systemic reactions on subsequent challenge by *S. invicta* to a lack of cross-sensitization between these two species of *Solenopsis*.

Case 5.—P. B. is a 31-year-old nonatopic male, a lifelong resident of Canada who had never been out of that country prior to 1972 when he visited Florida. While working under his car at the side of the road he sustained approximately 15 ant stings which produced pustules within 24 hours. Within a few minutes he developed generalized urticaria, angioedema, and wheezing. He collapsed and was cyanotic and unconscious on arrival at the emergency room in St. Petersburg, Florida. He responded to Epinephrine, intravenous steroids, oxygen, and Benadryl. He subsequently related that he had no known insect sensitivity and no previous ant sting reaction. He returned to Canada shortly after that without having been skin tested or treated. This case clearly could not have been the result of previous fire ant sensitization, and the sensitizing agent must have been some other insect with shared antigens.

A summary of the clinical cases previously documented in the literature is included (Table 10) (8, 59, 89, 91–98). Many of the cases in the literature are very poorly documented, frequently with no attempt to differentiate the type of ant involved. There are only three reports with good documentation of fire ant hypersensitivity including skin testing (91, 96, 99). The number of fairly well-documented cases in the literature is 37.

Triplett (99), in an unpublished survey, sent questionnaires to 2,485 doctors in 143 counties in Mississippi, Georgia, and Alabama, areas which were heavily infested with imported fire ants. He received replies from 1,325 of the doctors, who reported 9,422 patients in 1969, 11,937 in 1970, 12,438 in 1971. This survey was striking not only in its impressive reported trend of increased incidences over the 3-year period but also in the high number of secondary infection debridements, skin grafts, and a total of 19 cases of amputation. Of the total patients treated, approximately 10 percent (1,356 in 1971) were reported to have urticaria and/or angioedema with about half of these exhibiting other more serious signs of systemic involvement. A total of 154 cases of anaphylactic shock was reported and a total of 17 deaths. The estimated cost of medical care alone was over $350,000 for the year 1971.

Treatment Results

In Triplett's series (99), 8 of 18 patients on hyposensitization were re-stung by ants, which resulted in no systemic reactions. He could thus claim an apparent 100 percent therapy effectiveness. In our series, 19 of 92 patients treated were re-stung with 2 systemic reactions, producing, arithemetically at least, a 90 percent success

TABLE 10. Review of Literature

Author	Year	Cases	Comments
Caro: *Arch. Dermatol.* 75:475 (+ Discussion)	1957	3[c]	
		1 Death	No fire ant documentation
		2 General	No fire ant documentation
Thomas: *W. Va. Med. J.* 55:115	1959	1[b]	
Frazier: *Insect Allergy*	1969	1[a] Severe General	Frazier, in his book, refers to patient of Dr. Taylor's
Favorite: *Public Health Service Rep.* 73:445	1958	5[b] (2 Adult, 3 children)	
Helmly: *Hawaii Med. J.* 29:368	1970	1[b]	
Brown: *South. Med. J.* 65:273	1972	2[c]	
Micks: *Texas Rep. Biol. Med.* 18:624	1960	12[a]	5 Anaphylactic shock, no fire ant documentation
Triplett: *South. Med. J.* 66:477	1973	18[c]	Well-documented
Lockey: *J. Allergy Clin. Immunol.* 54:132	1974	2[c]	Well-documented
Olive: *J. Econ. Entomol.* 53:646	1960	5[b]	5 Systemic reactions in 300 cases of imported fire ant stings
Bowen: *South. Med. J.* 44:836	1951	1[a]	Patient died

a. No documentation that fire ant was offending species.
b. Clinical documentation of fire ant, i.e., pustule, ant identification, etc.
c. Clinical documentation + skin testing.

rate of therapy (Table 8). Triplett (100) has subsequently recorded 1 systemic reaction in a patient on immunotherapy. The difficulty of evaluating this data is demonstrated in Cases 3 and 4.

Case 2 did have a systemic reaction while well into hyposensitization. However, the patient had two subsequent re-stings with only local reactions, at even lower doses of extract. He, therefore, may not represent a treatment failure, although his course is difficult to explain. The patient J. B. (see Table 8) is also extremely interesting since in October of 1973, he was re-stung while receiving 1 to 1 thousand dilution and had only a local reaction. He was re-stung in April of 1974 and again in June of 1974 while receiving 1/2 cc of 1 to 1 thousand dilution and developed only a local reaction. In August of 1974 he was stung by 6 fire ants and experienced no difficulties; at that time he was almost at maintenance in his 1 to 10 dilution of extract. On August 16, he was stung by approximately 9 fire ants, and within an hour he began to experience severe itching of the hands, flushing of the face, tingling and numbness of the lips, and diplopia. He took 3 prednisone tablets, and the symptoms gradually began to subside. Although there were no objective signs, it was felt that this patient was not prone to hysteria. The reason for concern is that on theoretical grounds, we would expect to find individuals similar to those described by Lichtenstein, Valentine, and Sobotka (81) in cases of honeybee sensitivity, that is, certain patients who are sensitive only to components of the venom and who derive no protection from the commercial whole body extract.

There is one additional interesting patient not counted as a treatment failure who was mistakenly being treated with Greer red ant extract after a previous systemic reaction to fire ant and positive fire ant skin testing. On reexposure, she developed a systemic allergic reaction and was at that time started on fire ant extract. She has not been stung since.

Skin testing produces a number of false positives (8) and rare "false negatives" (see Table 4). Therefore, it is a helpful but not conclusive procedure.

There were 5 patients in the series, including Case 5, who had recently moved to the South from out of the country or from the northern United States, where they had lived all of their lives. With no known previous exposure, these 5 patients had systemic reactions to their first imported fire ant stings. This is strong evidence that they were initially sensitized through a cross-reacting antigen, probably from other insect exposures. This, together with the cases of individuals with combined hypersensitivity to the imported fire ant and other stinging hymenoptera, suggests, clinically at least, some cross-reaction.

The lack of systemic reaction on the subsequent sting (Case 3) demonstrates the variability of response even in a documented sensitive individual. In this case, with the short interval between episodes one might argue that he was stung during a "refractory period" and therefore did not react. This phenomenon of inconstant responses to subsequent challenges is seen fairly frequently in stinging hymenoptera sensitivity. This obviously makes claims of therapeutic success somewhat difficult to interpret. This claim is probably valid only if there have been multiple repeated exposures over a period of time without reaction. The apparent success rate of hyposensitization therapy remains impressive, however, in this limited number of 27 patients.

On the other side of this argument is the question of what percentage of patients who have already had one systemic allergic reaction to an ant sting will suffer a subsequent systemic reaction with a repeat sting. It is, of course, difficult or impossible to obtain this data. In our series of 104 patients, however, 19 gave a history of previous systemic reaction to ant stings. The majority of these reactions were progressively more severe and some became life-threatening. Most of these patients either did not realize the implications or the seriousness of the problem, or they did not realize that preventive treatment was available. Their histories demonstrate the possible dangers of not treating patients with systemic allergic reactions to fire ant stings.

The case for efficacy of immunotherapy with whole body extract of the imported fire ant is certainly far from proven. The weight of evidence currently available suggests that patients with more than the normal local reaction should at least be referred to an allergist for consideration of hyposensitization therapy.

Complications

Fire ant stings have been reported as a complication of alcoholism (90), which is not uncommon in certain areas (i.e., army installations). Complications of fire ant stings are, however, distinctly uncommon, with the exception of those noted in Triplett's survey (99).

Scarring (59), persistent nodules, and secondary eczematization (93) have been reported. Triplett (99) reports secondary infection and local necrosis requiring debridement and, in 19 cases, amputation. This is in sharp contrast to the experience of most allergists and other reports in the literature (89) in which secondary infection was rare and easily handled.

5
PREVENTION AND CONTROL

Control of the fire ant (101, 102) is inextricably tied to its fascinating and fickle political history. During the 1968 presidential campaign, Richard Nixon's campaign workers identified the fire ant as a uniquely southern problem, and in an attempt to woo the Southern vote, Nixon issued a statement promising "effective . . . control" of the imported fire ant. It was the first time many people in the North had ever heard of a fire ant. There was considerable local and regional interest in controlling this menace, and it was also at a time before environmentalism was in vogue. The history goes back even further. In the early 1950s, the South became well aware of the problem and struggled with it at the local level with no success. In 1958, help was demanded from Washington and \$2.4 million was appropriated for eradication. Along with this went an edict to the USDA to immediately eradicate the fire ant. A spraying program was hastily set up with the available chemicals heptachlor and dieldrin. The results were disastrous. A wide spectrum of insects, songbirds, raccoons, possums, quail, even cattle and turkeys, died. In response to this, Rachel Carson wrote *Silent Spring*. This book gave significant impetus to the development of the environmentalist movement.

The timing of this move was probably most unfortunate for the proponents of control programs, for not long after that field trials were begun on a new insecticide called Mirex (Fig. 15), developed by the Allied Chemical Company. It had been touted as the perfect insecticide, and there is significant basis for this claim. Although Mirex is toxic to many insects under laboratory conditions, it is highly selective when applied in the corncob grit and soybean oil bait used for ants. Markin (103) studied the effect of one Mirex application on the ant fauna of an area in Louisiana. He found that only certain species of ants were affected. The fire ants *S. invicta* and *S. xyloni* were reduced by 99 percent 1 week after aerial treatment. (The imported fire ant comprised 90 percent of the ant population prior to treatment.) Other ant species affected shared the characteristic of being primarily oil-preferring feeders. (Most of these species were considered to cause agricultural damage.) The sugar-feeding ant species were actually favored by the treatment since their numbers increased

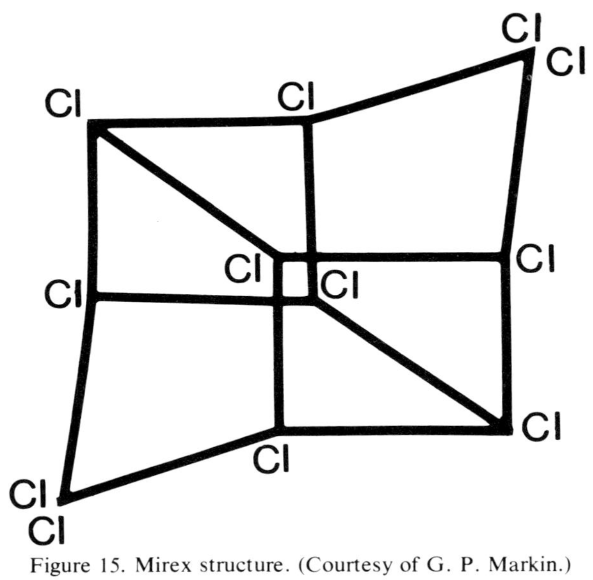

Figure 15. Mirex structure. (Courtesy of G. P. Markin.)

tenfold after the elimination of the fire ants. Good field trials with this agent have shown that aerial application of only 1.7 g of Mirex chemical in 1-1/4 lbs of corncob grit and soybean oil bait per acre is sufficient to eradicate over 95 percent of the fire ant population with one application (11, 103–5). Mirex not only kills the foraging workers, but also the workers in the nest, because it possesses delayed-action characteristics and the bait is brought back to the nest and consumed by the entire colony. A second application will result in almost complete eradication. Thus, we are talking about two thimblefuls of Mirex per acre. After treatment, the area will be reinfested within a few weeks via mating flights from surrounding areas (103). The imported fire ant population can be kept at acceptable levels by single aerial treatments every 12 months and, in some instances, as infrequently as every 3 years.

Mirex became available in time to fulfill Richard Nixon's 1968 campaign promise. It was applied aerially in poorly coordinated programs which were doomed to failure. Not all of the involved states participated in the 50-50 matching program with the federal government; thus, treated areas were quickly reinfested from untreated areas.

During this time, there was a steadily mounting pressure from the environmentalists, who equated the use of Mirex on the fire ant to "dropping nuclear bombs on pickpockets" (101). In the face of these complications, the USDA shifted its goal from a multiple spray eradication program covering the entire infected acreage (over 12 years at a cost of $200 million) to a spray program aimed at control of only 7 million acres (at a cost of $7 million by the year 1971). In spite of a clean bill of health given by a blue ribbon panel investigating the use and toxicity of Mirex, a court injunction was issued banning the aerial application of the chemical. This restriction crippled the truly effective use of Mirex.

Another political turn which has not helped the Mirex cause was the observation that the main Allied Chemical plant involved in the production of Mirex bait is located in Mississippi, and the congressional committee which appropriated the fire ant money had very strong Mississippi representation. Much political hay was made of this, but analysis of the facts indicates this was probably not a significant relationship.

To further complicate the issue, more recent information indicates that under certain nonphysiologic conditions fish kills have resulted from the use of Mirex. In addition, a 1969 panel of the Department of Health, Education, and Welfare classified Mirex as a potential carcinogen and recommended limited use (101). There is, however, no evidence to confirm this in any sort of realistic exposures.

In any event, Mirex is highly selective (for an insecticide) for many ant species, including fire ants. It is by far the most effective control method currently available. It was generally available through county agents or from Allied Chemical Company and can be applied in very small amounts in the corncob bait to a backyard area or in the treatment of farm acreage. Intermittent application can give good control of small areas, and thus far there is no evidence of resistance on the part of the fire ant.

The USDA aerial treatment program treated 12 million acres in 8 states during 1974 and was effective in control. However, the program is still under attack in current EPA hearings into Mirex. The weight of evidence is in favor of Mirex as a safe and effective control (not eradicator) of the imported fire ant. The USDA did not await the outcome of the hearings but discontinued the aerial spraying program, reportedly due to EPA restrictions which the USDA felt made the program ineffective. Subsequently, Allied Chemical stopped production of the Mirex bait, and the product is no longer available; this leaves little relief for the homeowner and farmer.

The most recent information available on the status of Mirex is contained in *Environmental News* of May 7, 1976, published by the Environmental Protection Agency. The state of Mississippi has recently decided to purchase from Allied Chemical Corporation the only Mirex production plant in the U.S., which is located at Aberdeen Prairie, Mississippi. It is anticipated that enough Mirex bait will be produced to allow aerial treatment of 5 million acres in Mississippi, Alabama, Arkansas, Florida, Georgia, Louisiana, North Carolina, South Carolina, and Texas during 1976. The same restrictions will apply, namely one application per year with no aerial treatment of areas near major bodies of water or forested areas. These are the same restrictions to which the USDA objected when it withdrew from the application program. This year it will be done by involved states.

In addition, a new bait formulation called 10:5 has been used in field trials in Florida, Georgia, and Mississippi and has been shown to be as effective as the current Mirex in controlling fire ants, but it contains about 75 percent less Mirex per treated acre. This should further diminish concerns over environmental hazards. Further experiments are being carried out to determine what frequency of application of the new bait results in maximal suppression of the fire ant population. According to a letter from J. R. Quarrles, Deputy Administrator of EPA, if it is demonstrated that "multiple applications would decrease the rate of infestation without posing a proportionally greater environmental risk . . .

this . . . could lead to a modification of the present restrictions on aerial broadcast applications to allow up to three uses of 10:5 in a two year period.''

A press release of July 1976, reporting the finding of Mirex in a significant number of human tissue samples surveyed has not yet altered the official policy on the insecticide. These data are the first clear indictment of Mirex as a possible hazard to humans. They greatly cloud the already uncertain future of the chemical.

Certainly, fire ants are sensitive to chlordane, dieldrin (removed from the market as a carcinogen), and some of the other common insecticides. However, these are not nearly as effective as Mirex and require direct application and direct contact; furthermore, it is unlikely that even correct application and drowning of the colony will result in its eradication. The only good relief for the homeowner at the present time is Mirex.

Avoidance is the best treatment of all, when feasible. Unfortunately, this is frequently difficult, especially in the case of children. The desirability of wearing shoes and long pants and staying away from known infested areas are frequently forgotten admonitions in the case of playing children. We have certainly seen many instances in which the sensitive child, and even the adult, was re-stung on numerous occasions while repeating the same activity which had gotten him into trouble before.

In spite of the efficacy of Mirex, it is certainly not the ultimate answer, because of possible toxicity, cost of application, and the necessity for repeated application. There is currently great interest in natural control mechanisms. Allen and Buren have found protozoa of the genus *Thelohania* in *S. invicta* specimens obtained from the Mato Grosso area (106). Currently, protozoa of the genus *Nosema* are being used in control of the grasshopper in the western United States, and some control has been attained with mosquitoes as well. Virus-like particles have been found by electron microscopy in some fire ant specimens from South America, and this might offer a very promising solution (106). Natural enemies of *S. invicta* include the army ant, anteaters, and certain parasitic ants; however, these are not realistic controls since the "cure" might be worse than the "disease."

Another avenue of investigation is the juvenile hormone. This is a normal insect hormone, but synthetic analogues (methoprene and hydroprene) can cause maturational arrest of larvae and temporary sterility (11). Further, inhibition and death of the imported fire ant colonies have also been achieved with the feeding of insect growth regulators, another group of insect hormones, in doses of 5 mg per colony (107).

Three species of fungi (i.e., *Aspergillus flavus*) and a *Pseudomonas* species have been shown to be pathogenic to *S. invicta* and *S. richteri* and are being currently investigated (11). It is not clear whether this represents a natural control mechanism, but it is being studied with great interest. A parasite would certainly potentially serve as an ideal natural control agent which would have extreme specificity and would require only one introduction into a given area. Other factors being studied in the Mato Grosso field station include the effects of temperature, rainfall, parasites, predators, competing species, etc., in the control of the distribution of *S. invicta*.

The USDA has received a great deal of bad press over this issue, and there is a certain degree of fatalism which now prevails concerning the fire ant problem. It is probably the new awareness of the increasing population at risk to anaphylactic reaction from fire ant stings that may help spur further interest in control mechanisms.

REFERENCES

1. Clausen, L. W.: *Insect Fact and Folklore*. New York: Macmillan, 1954, pp. 107–16.
2. Rhoades, R. B., Schafer, W. L., Schmid, W. H., Wubbena, P. F., Dozier, R. M., Townes, A. W., and Wittig, H. J.: Hypersensitivity to the imported fire ant. A report of 49 cases. *J. Allergy Clin. Immunol.* 56:84, 1975.
3. Wilson, E. O.: *The Insect Societies*. Cambridge: Harvard University Press, 1971.
4. Wilson, E. O.: A report on the imported fire ant, *Solenopsis saevissima richteri*, in Alabama. Special Report to the Alabama Department of Conservation, 1949.
5. Wilson, E. O.: Enemy specification in the alarm-recruitment system of an ant. *Science* 190:798, 1975.
6. Whitcomb, J. H.: Personal communication, 1976.
7. Buren, W. F.: Personal communication, 1975.
8. Lockey, R. F.: Systemic reactions to stinging ants. *J. Allergy Clin. Immunol.* 54:132, 1974.
9. Parrish, H. M.: Analysis of 460 fatalities from venomous animals in the United States. *Am. J. Med. Sci.* 245:129, 1963.
10. Pinnas, J. L., Wang, T. M., Strunk, R. C., and Thompson, H. C.: Harvester ant hypersensitivity; in vitro and in vivo studies. *J. Allergy Clin. Immunol.* 55:107, 1975.
11. Lofgren, C. S.: Biology and control of imported fire ants. *Ann. Rev. Entomol.* 20:1, 1975.
12. Jouvenaz, D. P., and Adams, C. T.: Personal communication, 1975.
13. Buren, W. F.: Zoogeography of the imported fire ants. *J. N.Y. Entomol. Soc.* 82:113, 1974.
14. Markin, G. P., Dillier, J. H., and Collins, H. L.: Growth and development of colonies of the red imported fire ant, *Solenopsis invicta*. *Ann. Entomol. Soc. Am.* 66:803, 1973.
15. A survey of the economic impact of the imported fire ant on farmers in the southern United States. Chilton Research Services, October 1973 (unpublished work).
16. *Yearbook of Agriculture*. United States Department of Agriculture, 1952, p. 468.
17. Buren, W. F.: Revisionary studies on the taxonomy of the imported fire ants. *J. Georgia Entomol. Soc.* 7:1, 1972.
18. Brand, J. M., Blum, M. S., and Barlin, M. R.: Fire ant venoms: Intraspecific and interspecific variation among castes and individuals. *Toxicon* 11:325, 1973.

19. Markin, G. P., Collins, H. L., and Dillier, J. H.: Colony founding by queens of the red imported fire ant, *Solenopsis invicta*. *Ann. Entomol. Soc. Am.* 65:1053, 1972.
20. Rhoades, W. C., and Davis, D. R.: Effects of meteorologic factors on the biology and control of the imported fire ant. *J. Econ. Entomol.* 6:554, 1967.
21. Forbes, J.: The anatomy and histology of the male reproductive system of *Camponotus pennsylvanicus* DeGeer (Formicidae, Hymenoptera). *J. Morphol.* 95:523, 1954.
22. Markin, G. P., Dillier, J. H., Hill, S. O., Blum, M. S., and Hermann, H. R.: Nuptial flight and flight ranges of the imported fire ant, *Solenopsis saevissima richteri* (Hymenoptera: Formicidae). *J. Georgia Entomol. Soc.* 6:145, 1971.
23. Lofgren, C. S.: On the eradication of imported fire ants: A theoretical appraisal. *Bull. Entomol. Soc. Am.* 18:17, 1972.
24. Brian, M. V.: Caste determination in a Myrmicine ant. *Experientia* 7:182, 1951.
25. Sisson, R. F.: At home with the bulldog ant. *National Geographic* (July):62, 1974.
26. Peacock, A. D.: Studies in Pharaoh's ant, *Monomorium pharaonis*. *Entomologists Monthly Magazine* 86:171, 1950.
27. Von Hagen, V. W.: The ant that carries a parasol. *Natural History* 43:27, 1939.
28. Martin, M. M., and Weber, N. A.: *In* Wilson, E. O.: *The Insect Societies*. Cambridge: Harvard University Press, 1971.
29. Weber, N. A.: Weeding as a factor in fungus culture by ants. *Anat. Rec.* 128:638, 1957.
30. Stahel, G., and Geijskes, D. C.: Von *Atta Cephalotes* L. and *Atta Serdens*. *Rev. Entomol.* (*Rio de Janeiro*) 10:27, 1939.
31. Janzen, D. H.: Allelopathy by Myrmecophytes: The ant azteca as an allelopathic agent of *Cecropia*. *Ecology* 50:147, 1969.
32. Wheeler, W. M.: *Ants: Their Structure, Development and Behavior*. New York: Columbia University Press, 1960.
33. Schneirla, T. C.: Basic correlations and coordinations in insect societies with special reference to ants. *Colloq. Intern. Centre Nat. Rech. Sci.* (*Paris*) 34:247, 1950.
34. Wheeler, W. M.: The physiognomy of insects. *Quart. Rev. Biol.* 2:1, 1927.
35. Creighton, W. S.: The habits of *Pheidole multicida* Wheeler. *Psyche* 66:1, 1959.
36. Eible-Eibesfeldt, I., and Eible-Eibesfeldt, E.: Das parasitenabwehren der minima-arbeiterinnen der blattschneiderameise, *Atta cephalotes*. *Z. Tierpsychol.* 24:278, 1967.
37. v. Frish, K.: Die polarisation des himmelslichtes als orientierender faktor bei den tänzen der bienen. *Experientia* 5:142, 1949.
38. Vowles, D. M.: The orientation of ants. 2. Orientation to light, gravity and polarized light. *J. Exp. Biol.* 31:356, 1954.
39. Werringloer, A.: Die sehorgane und sehzentren der dorylinen nebst untersuchunger uber die facettenaugen der formiciden. *Z. Wiss. Zool.* (*Abt. A*) 141:432, 1932.
40. Vass, C.: Uber das formensehen der roten waldameise (*Formica rufa-gruppe*). *Z. Vergleich. Physiol.* 55:255, 1967.
41. Marak, G. E., and Wolken, J. J.: An action spectrum for fire ant, *Solenopsis saevissima*. *Nature* 205:1328, 1965.

42. Wilson, E. O.: Chemical communication among workers of the fire ant, *Solenopsis saevissima* (Fr. Smith). 1. The organization of mass-foraging. *Anim. Behav.* 10:134, 1962.
43. Brun, R.: *Die Raumorientierung der Ameisen und das Orientierungsproblem im Allgemeinen*. Jena: Gustav Fischer, 1914, 8, p. 234.
44. Jander, R.: Die optische richtungsorientierung der roten waldameise. *Z. Vergleich. Physiol.* 40:162, 1957.
45. Wilson, E. O.: Chemical systems. *In* Sebeok, T. A. (ed.): *Animal Communication, Techniques of Study and Results of Research*. Bloomington: Indiana University Press, 1968, p. 75.
46. Blum, M. S.: Personal communication, 1975.
47. Möglich, M., Maschwitz, U., and Hölldobler, B.: Tandem calling: A new kind of signal in ant communication. *Science* 186:1046, 1974.
48. Hangartner, W.: Spezifitat und inaktivierung des spurpheromones von lasius fuliginosus. *Z. Vergleich. Physiol.* 57:103, 1967.
49. Lindauer, M.: *Communication among Social Bees*. Cambridge: Harvard University Press, 1961, p. 143.
50. Jouvenaz, D. P.: Fire ants: Attraction of workers to queen secretions. *Ann. Entomol. Soc. Am.* 67:442, 1974.
51. Wilson, E. O.: Chemical communication in the social insects. *Science* 149:1064, 1965.
52. Stratton, L. O., and Coleman, W. P.: Maze learning and orientation in the fire ant, *Solenopsis saevissima*. *J. Comp. Physiol. Psychol.* 83:7, 1973.
53. Chauvin, R.: Experiences sur l'apprentissage par equipe du labyrinthe chez *Formica polyctena*. *Insectes Sociaux* 11:1, 1964.
54. Jander, R.: Die optische richtung-sorientierung der roten waldameise (*F. rufa*). *Z. Vergleich. Physiol.* 49:162, 1957.
55. Thorpe, W. H., and Zangwill, O. L.: *Current Problems in Animal Behavior*. London: Cambridge University Press, 1961, pp. 5–29.
56. Russell, F. E.: Venomous animal injuries. *Curr. Probl. Pediatr.* 3, 1973.
57. Minton, S. A.: Snake venoms and envenomation (Editorial). *Clin. Toxicol.* 3:343, 1970.
58. Habermann, E.: Bee and wasp venoms. *Science* 177:314, 1972.
59. Caro, M. R., Derbes, V. J., and Jung, R.: Skin responses to the sting of the imported fire ant, *Solenopsis saevissima*. *Arch. Dermatol.* 75:475, 1957.
60. Adrouny, G. A., Derbes, V. J., and Jung, R. C.: Isolation of a hemolytic component of fire ant venom. *Science* 130:449, 1959.
61. Jung, R. C.: Skin response to solamine, a hemolytic component of fire ant venom. *Dermatologia Tropica* 5:241, 1964.
62. Blum, M. S., Walker, J. R., Callahan, P. S., and Novak, A. F.: Chemical, insecticidal, and antibiotic properties of fire ant venom. *Science* 128:306, 1958.
63. Quarterly report, USDA (Mississippi), 1973.
64. Blum, M. S.: Chemistry of the venom of *Solenopsis aurea*. *Ann. Entomol. Soc. Am.* 66:702, 1973.
65. MacConnell, J. G., Blum, M. S., and Fales, H. M.: Alkaloid from fire ant venom: Identification and synthesis. *Science* 168:840, 1970.
66. Brand, J. M., Blum, M. S., Fales, H. M., and MacConnell, J. G.: Fire ant venoms: Comparative analysis of alkaloidal components. *Toxicon* 10:259, 1972.
67. Brand, J. M., and Blum, M. S.: Biochemical evolution in fire ant venoms. *Insect Biochem.* 3:34, 1973.
68. Buffkin, D. C.: Some chemical and pharmacologic properties of the venom of the imported fire ant, *Solenopsis saevissima richteri*. *Tier-und Pflanzengifte*, 1972.

69. Jouvenaz, D. P., Blum, M. S., and MacConnell, J. G.: Antibacterial activity of venom alkaloids from the imported fire ant, *Solenopsis invicta* Buren. *Antimicrob. Agents Chemother.* 2:291, 1972.

70. Buffkin, D. C., and Russell, F. E.: Some chemical and pharmacological properties of the venom of the imported fire ant, *Solenopsis saevissima richteri*. *Toxicon* 10:526, 1972.

71. Narahashi, T.: In letter to M. S. Blum, 1974.

72. Hoffman, E.: Personal communication, 1975.

73. Ishizaka, K.: Experimental anaphylaxis. *In* Samter, M. (ed.): *Immunological Diseases*. Boston: Little Brown and Company, 1971, p. 206.

74. Foubert, E. L., and Stier, R. A.: Antigenic relationships between honeybees, wasps, yellow hornets, black hornets, and yellow jackets. *J. Allergy* 29:13, 1958.

75. Langlois, C., Shulman, S., Kozmycz, S., and Arbesman, C. E.: The allergic response to stinging insects. 6. Fractionation of whole body and venom sac extracts of wasp. *J. Allergy* 37:359, 1966.

76. Arbesman, C. E., Langlois, C., and Shulman, S.: The allergic response to stinging insects. 4. Cross-reactions between bee, wasp, and yellow jacket. *J. Allergy* 36:147, 1965.

77. Shulman, S., Bigelsen, F., Lang, R., and Arbesman, C.: The allergic response to stinging insects: Biochemical and immunologic studies on bee venom and other bee body preparations. *J. Immunol.* 96:29, 1966.

78. Arbesman, C. E., Langlois, C., Bronsra, P., and Shulman, S.: The allergic response to stinging insects. 7. Fractionation of whole body and venom sac extracts of yellow jacket. *J. Allergy* 38:1, 1966.

79. Barr, S. E.: Allergy to hymenoptera stings—Review of the world literature. *Ann. Allergy* 29:49, 1971.

80. O'Connor, R., and Erickson, R.: Hymenoptera antigens: An immunological comparison of venoms, venom sac extracts and whole-insect extracts. *Ann. Allergy* 23:151, 1965.

81. Lichtenstein, L. M., Valentine, M. D., and Sobotka, A. K.: A case for venom treatment in anaphylactic sensitivity to hymenoptera sting. *N. Engl. J. Med.* 290:1223, 1974.

82. Loveless, M. H.: Immunization in wasp sting allergy through venom repositories and periodic insect stings. *J. Immunol.* 89:204, 1962.

83. Insect sting allergy: Questionnaire study of 2606 cases. *JAMA* 193:115, 1965.

84. Spence, J. E.: A comparison of the allergenic and immunological effects of the hemolytic component of fire ant venom. *Tulane University of Louisiana Medical School Prize Essay* 7:212, 1962–63.

85. Buren, W. F.: The widespread occurrence of mandibular grooves in aculeate hymenoptera. *J. Georgia Entomol. Soc.* 5:185, 1970.

86. James, F., Pence, H. L., Driggers, D. P., Jacobs, R. L., and Horton, D. E.: In vivo and in vitro studies of human reactions to fire ant venom. *J. Allergy Clin. Immunol.* (Abstr.) 57:209, 1976.

87. Blum, M. S., Roberts, J. E., Jr., and Novak, A. F.: Chemical and biological characteristics of venom of the ant *Solenopsis Xyloni* McCook. *Psyche* 68:73, 1961.

88. Rhoades, R. B., Schafer, W. L., Newman, M., Lockey, R., Dozier, R. M., Wubbena, P. F., Townes, A. W., Schmid, W. H., Neder, G., Brill, T., and Wittig, H. J.: Hypersensitivity to the imported fire ant in Florida. A report of 104 cases. (In preparation.)

89. Olive, A. T.: Infestation of the imported fire ant, *Solenopsis saevissima richteri*, at Fort Benning, Georgia. *J. Econ. Entomol.* 53:646, 1960.

90. Smith, J. D., and Smith, E. B.: Multiple fire ant stings. A complication of alcoholism. *Arch. Dermatol.* 103:438, 1971.
91. Triplett, R. F.: Sensitivity to the imported fire ant: Successful treatment with immunotherapy. *South. Med. J.* 66:477, 1973.
92. Thomas, J. W.: Allergic reactions following insect bites and stings and their management. *W. Virginia Med. J.* 55:115, 1959.
93. Frazier, C. A.: *Insect Allergy: Allergic Reactions to Bites of Insects and Other Arthropods.* St. Louis, Mo.: W. H. Green, Inc., 1969.
94. Favorite, F. G.: The imported fire ant. *Public Health Service Rep.* 73:445, 1958.
95. Helmly, R. B.: Anaphylactic reaction to fire ant. *Hawaii Med. J.* 29:368, 1970.
96. Brown, L. L.: Fire ant allergy. *South. Med. J.* 65:273, 1972.
97. Micks, D. W.: Insects and other arthropods of medical importance in Texas. *Texas Rep. Biol. Med.* 18:624, 1960.
98. Bowen, R. B.: Insects and allergic problems. *South. Med. J.* 44:836, 1951.
99. Triplett, R. F.: Questionnaire survey (unpublished work).
100. Triplett, R. F.: Personal communication, 1974.
101. Shapley, D.: Mirex and the fire ant: Decline in fortunes of "perfect" pesticide. *Science* 172:358, 1971.
102. Ferguson, D. E.: Fire ant: Whose pest? *Science* 169:630, 1970.
103. Markin, G. P.: Effects of Mirex on the general ant fauna of a treated area in Louisiana (unpublished work).
104. Stringer, C. E.: Imported fire ant toxic bait studies: Evaluation of toxicants. *J. Econ. Entomol.* 57:941, 1964.
105. Lofgren, C. S.: Imported fire ant toxic bait studies: Further tests with granulated Mirex—soybean oil bait. *J. Econ. Entomol.* 57:695, 1964.
106. Allen, G. E., and Buren, W. F.: Microsporidan and fungal diseases of *Solenopsis invicta* Buren in Brazil. *J. N.Y. Entomol. Soc.* 82:125, 1974.
107. Vinson, S. B., and Robeau, R.: Insect growth regulator effects on colonies of the imported fire ant. *J. Econ. Entomol.* 67:584, 1974.